Penguin Books

35 mm Dreams

Sue Mathews was born in Melbourne in 1952. She was at
Monash University from 1970 to 1974, where she
completed an honours degree in sociology, and edited the
student newspaper *Lot's Wife* in her final year. She joined
the Australian Broadcasting Commission in 1975, and
worked as a radio producer in Brisbane and Melbourne.
An interest in radio that combined ideas with popular
music was consolidated when in 1977 she was appointed
manager of 3RRR–FM, Melbourne's educational public
broadcasting radio station. She lived in New York for a
year in 1981, working as a freelance writer and radio
producer. Most recently she has produced a series of radio
programs on Australian movies for American public radio.

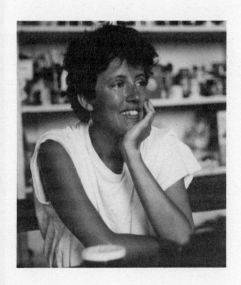

3 5 mm DREAMS

Sue Mathews

PENGUIN BOOKS

Penguin Books Australia Ltd,
487 Maroondah Highway, P.O. Box 257
Ringwood, Victoria, 3134, Australia
Penguin Books Ltd,
Harmondsworth, Middlesex, England
Penguin Books,
40 West 23rd Street, New York, N.Y. 10010, U.S.A.
Penguin Books Canada Ltd,
2801 John Street, Markham, Ontario, Canada
Penguin Books (N.Z.) Ltd,
182–190 Wairau Road, Auckland 10, New Zealand

First published by Penguin Books Australia, 1984

Copyright © Sue Mathews, 1984

Typeset in Clearface by Dudley E. King, Melbourne

Made and printed in Australia by
Dominion Press–Hedges and Bell

CIP

Mathews, Sue, 1952– .
35 mm dreams.

Includes index.
ISBN 0 14 006709 4.

1. Moving-picture producers and directors –
Australia – Interviews. I. Title.

791.43′0233′0922

CONTENTS

ACKNOWLEDGEMENTS

I must thank Bob Ellis (for suggesting that this book be written), Peter Hamilton (for helping lay much of the groundwork) and Andrew Houlding (for encouraging – and publishing – some of my early writing on Australian movies). For ideas about film and popular culture in general, I should thank Robert Jordan and Greig Pickhaver for many hours of conversation and inspiration.

Kerry Conway, Uri Windt and Sue Murray made very helpful suggestions about the introduction. Bruce Sims from Penguin helped devise the book and shape the interviews, Margaret Eliot typed the transcripts and Tim Fraser did a tactful and intelligent job of editing the manuscript.

And for support and encouragement, both professional and emotional, through the book's history and a lot else besides, thanks to my parents Rivkah and Bob Mathews and my friend Mark Burford.

INTRODUCTION

'There were no chases in *Mad Max*,' says director George Miller. 'We didn't stage a chase up at Broken Hill. Chases are little pieces of film put together in a movie theatre. The drama happens in the audience's mind.'

Every year 55 million cinema tickets are bought in Australia. In those figures, four times a year each Australian pays seven dollars to go to the pictures. Sitting in the dark in a movie theatre a film appears to us as a fait accompli. We can take it or leave it as we respond to the experience it gives us of amusement, enlightenment, or, to quote George Miller again, a feeling like being 'on a roller-coaster ride'. But if there are no chases in *Mad Max*, no mystery at *Hanging Rock*, no love affair in *My Brilliant Career*, what is it we are watching?

Each of the 24 frames per second that go to make up a movie is part of a process. A movie is the outcome of countless decisions made by a wide range of people with a very diverse set of interests. They include directors and writers and cameramen making decisions about how a story will be turned into moving images; accountants and investors making decisions about risks and profits; unions making decisions about conditions under which people will record the sound, load the clapperboards, do the stunts; distributors making decisions about which films are most likely to attract the seven-dollar customers; and in many parts of the world key decisions are made by politicians and public servants concerned to promote a sense of national identity and pride.

Fifteen years ago the idea that there could be a book about a group of directors in Australia who between them had made 25 feature films would have seemed preposterous. That is part of the story this book will tell. These interviews are a series of portraits of five creative film directors; together they make up a portrait of the new Australian cinema. The first section of each interview, 'Beginnings', tells how

1

each director's career merged with the development of the new Australian cinema. The second part, 'Making the Movies', deals with how and why each film came to be made and how it was put together. In the third part, 'Reflecting on Directing', some more general issues which confront the film director are raised, from the place of politics in movie making to the practical problems of being a first-time director. The final section of each interview, except Peter Weir's, looks at the qualities that give the Australian cinema its distinctive character and asks whether Australian directors will continue to develop a national cinema or move into an international arena based in Hollywood.

In the years between 1942 and 1969, almost no Australian feature films were produced. In the next decade over 200 features appeared that had been produced, directed and written by Australians. You could be forgiven for thinking that the entire Australian film industry sprang into being by spontaneous generation at the sound of the words, 'This Bill provides for the establishment of an Australian Film Development Corporation ... to encourage the production and distribution of Australian films of high quality', spoken by the then Prime Minister John Gorton in 1970. Of course, it wasn't quite like that – and these five interviews provide five different perspectives on the question of where the Australian cinema did come from.

John Gorton was certainly an idiosyncratic Liberal Prime Minister, a man with a larrikin, almost Rabelaisian, style. His decision to establish an Australian Film Development Corporation to fund and promote a national film industry came in response to intense lobbying from several Australian critics and would-be film producers. Among them were Sylvia Lawson, Colin Bennett and Michael Thornhill. Closest to Gorton's ear were Phillip Adams, the irreverent advertising executive, newspaper columnist and soon-to-be film producer (who in 1983 was appointed as Chairman of the Australian Film Commission), and Barry Jones, former star of the television quiz show *Pick-a-Box*, a Labor Party MP who in 1983 became Minister for Science and Technology. There had been eighteen years of profoundly conservative rule by Prime Minister Sir Robert Menzies, who had kept a firm clamp on government expenditure on indulgences like the arts, and Gorton, a most unlikely inheritor of Menzies' mantle, appears in contrast as a latter-day Medici presiding over a cultural renaissance. The Gorton era saw the establishment of the Australian Council for the Arts (now the Australia Council) to promote all aspects of the arts in Australia as well as the birth of the new film industry.

Many things were changing in Australia in 1970 and the encouragement by government of an indigenous culture reflected movement in many quarters. That year saw some of the biggest mass demonstrations in Australia's history, with over 130 000 people marching down Bourke Street in Melbourne and blocking streets surrounding Sydney's Town Hall, demanding an end to Australia's involvement in the Vietnam War. When President Lyndon Johnson visited Australia in 1966 he was greeted by a Prime Minister proclaiming an Australian foreign policy of 'All The Way With LBJ'. But within three or four years the dependent stance in foreign policy was being dramatically challenged. Along with that rejection came a re-examination of Australia's dependent stance in just about everything, from exploitation of the country's natural resources to the images and values absorbed from television, popular music, and the movies.

Cultural dependence was a habit Australians had found hard to break, from the time of the country's colonisation by upwardly mobile working-class and lower-middle-class settlers from the British Isles in the nineteenth century. Right up until the fifties you could hear second and even third-generation Australians refer to England as 'home'. Anything English was judged worthy, valuable, refined, while things Australian were rough, crude, second best. Even after the colonial ties to England had frayed beyond repair, the concern with propriety and sobriety remained a powerful force in Australia – in 1983 Australia's censorship laws remain tighter than in almost any other Western country, and in many cities it is impossible to purchase alcohol after ten o'clock at night.

But there has been another equally persistent strand in the culture. Alongside the Australian incarnation of the proper gentleman there has been a popular image of the (usually male) Australian as the bushman; the cocky, or small farmer; or the miner. The roots of this tradition probably lie less in the would-be gentry who came to Australia after the 1840s than in the Irish who became the rebels of the Australian goldfields in the 1860s and in those who preceded them all, the convicts for whose safe and remote detention the English had originally established the colony. The image is of the ordinary bloke, the battler; always the soldier, never the officer. His qualities of egalitarianism, scepticism, humour and low tolerance of pretension had been a feature of popular literature and cartoons since the end of the last century, and they were crystallised in the World War One image of the Anzacs, the soldiers who fought at Gallipoli in 1915.

The nationalist arguments for an Australian film industry had something for everyone, as would the films themselves. To those concerned with respectability and still plagued by feelings of inferiority it was argued that a film industry turning out serious reflections on Australian life, which also touched on universal themes, would generate respect and recognition from our international elders and betters. And to those who valued a more rebellious national feeling it offered the chance to assert positively what was distinctive about Australia and Australians, as an antidote to the colonisation of Australian hearts and minds by England and America.

The nationalist arguments were strengthened by the rediscovery of a genuine Australian film tradition. The unearthing of a history that became even more glorious in the telling helped the lobbyists establish the existence of both a long-forgotten attraction of Australian audiences to Australian films and a lineage of Australians who had distinguished themselves as producers, directors and stars of the silver screen. The explanation given for the demise of that tradition was strangulation by foreign predators, made possible by the passivity of Australian businessmen interested in a fast buck and Australian governments interested in an easy life. The setting up of a new Australian cinema became almost the patriotic duty of a self-respecting contemporary Australian government.

The original Australian film industry had indeed played a pioneering role in world cinema. As early as 1896 short films were being made around Melbourne and shown as part of variety reviews in live theatre. In 1900 a feature-length film and slide show named *Soldiers of the Cross* was made by the Salvation Army in the grounds of a home for wayward girls. It had Christians, lions, and legions of Roman soldiers, and aspired to all the grandeur and excess that became characteristic of the de Mille epics years later. *The Story of the Kelly Gang,* an 80-minute film made by Charles Tait in 1906 is reputed to have been the world's first feature-length production, and it established a precedent for Australian films about Australian subjects achieving real popularity with Australian audiences. Other bushranging tales followed, as well as melodramas and historical romances. Despite fluctuations, Australia had a productive, profitable, and sophisticated film industry.

In the following years many films were made, including several that would attain the status of classics in the pantheon erected by the film lobbyists of the sixties – Raymond Longford's *The Sentimental Bloke* (1919) and *On Our Selection* (1920) were high on the list. Australians were avid movie goers: in 1920 the total attendance was 67.5 million, which was more than ten times the population of the country. But attendance figures like that were too good to be ignored by the burgeoning Hollywood movie industry, and several American production companies set up distribution offices in Australia, while other American firms bought and built cinemas in Australia that were as grand as the movie palaces of Hollywood itself. The Hollywood studios, with their huge advantages of scale and capital, were beginning to outstrip other industries with larger and more lavish productions and vigorous overseas marketing operations.

During the 1920s the creation of the Hoyts theatre chain, which was American-controlled after 1930 (and would remain so until 1982), made significant inroads into the field of exhibition which until then had been dominated by the local Union theatres. Union theatres had been formed in 1913 as the exhibition wing of the distributor Australasian Films, setting the pattern for the linking of exhibition and distribution that has been accepted in Australia ever since. A 50 per cent interest in this group of companies, by then known as Greater Union, was sold to the British film production company Rank soon after World War Two. But long before then the plentiful supply of films whose production costs had been met by overseas studios, and whose marketability had been tested by overseas audiences, made it good business sense for distributors and exhibitors to concentrate on foreign product. As a consequence, Australian producers found it harder and harder to find outlets for their films, or finance for production.

But the greatest single blow to the early Australian industry was dealt by the advent of the talkies. Like the industries of France and England, the Australian film industry was swamped. And like the Europeans they lacked the resources to develop any real challenge to the big, flashy talking pictures that issued from Hollywood following *The Jazz Singer* (1927), when people gasped as they first watched Al Jolson's gesticulations and heard him singing at the same time. The idea of an 'economic conspiracy' as the basic for the demise of the Australian film industry is downplayed by David Williams, General Manager of the Greater Union Organisation. 'The Americans didn't set out to crush the Australian industry,' he says, 'they didn't have to. When you had something like Garbo in *Flesh and the Devil* up on the screen, an Australian film just couldn't compete.'

During the thirties, feature production in Australia was reduced to the province of one organisation: Cinesound, the studio set up by Greater Union in 1931. Cinesound was managed, and most of its films were directed, by Ken G. Hall. There were some outstanding successes, including a remake of *On Our Selection* (1931), based on Steele Rudd's story of the pioneer country bumpkins Dad and Dave, and *The Squatter's Daughter,* a romantic adventure film on a sheepstation featuring raging bushfires and 10 000 sheep. While many of the topics were Australian, Hall's approach and style drew heavily on Hollywood. Cinesound had an extraordinary success ratio – of seventeen films released, sixteen returned a profit. Despite this the new regime at Greater Union following the merger with Rank deemed local film production a non-commercial proposition. Cinesound's feature production facilities were closed permanently after World War Two, although the organisation continued to function as a producer of newsreels to be screened before the main feature at Greater Union theatres. The camera crew shown in Phillip Noyce's *Newsfront* (1978) rowing open dinghies through torrential floodwaters and mending broken axles in rugged desert car rallies is loosely based on the Cinesound newsreel team.

The newsreels were among the few small pockets of filmmaking skills kept alive after the war. They owed their existence to government support: they were the one concession made by exhibitors to the Cinematographic Act of 1935 which laid down an Australian content quota for cinemas in New South Wales. But whatever real teeth that Act may have had at its inception were quickly drawn, and no requirement to provide Australian feature films was ever enforced. That Australia's links with Britain were still enormously powerful is indicated by the pressure for the establishment of an 'Empire quota', and the resultant proviso that protection of Australian films must never be at the expense of British films, which were shielded in Australia from American competition.

The extinguishing of the Cinesound arc lights signalled thirty years in which Charles Chauvel's wartime productions *Forty Thousand Horsemen* (1940) and *The Rats of Tobruk* (1944), his *Sons of Matthew* (1949) and *Jedda* (1957), and Cecil Holmes' *Three in One* (1957) were the only fully Australian films produced. Australia's contribution to world cinema consisted of providing a back lot for a handful of American and British productions. One such film was *On the Beach* (1959), adapted from the novel by Nevil Shute. It was a story about survivors of a nuclear holocaust, and when its star, Ava Gardner, told the press that she thought Melbourne was 'a dump' and a very suitable location for a movie about the end of the world, many Australians still in the grip of the cultural cringe probably concurred. The existence of an Australian film industry had sunk from memory, leaving not even a glimmer of possibility. Movie attendances remained high, but except for a few filmmaking die-hards the notion that good films might actually be made in Australia had receded beyond the limits of imagination.

In fact it was theatre rather than movies that was the site of the first visible reassertion of nationalism in Australian culture. John Duigan describes new movements in Melbourne theatre in the late sixties; in Sydney there was parallel activity. Peter Weir recalls the impact of shows like *The Legend of King O'Malley*, a satirical portrait of the politician who founded Canberra, the national capital. One of *King O'Malley's* authors was Bob Ellis, now a noted film scriptwriter; another leading screenwriter is the acclaimed playwright David Williamson, co-writer of Peter Weir's *Gallipoli* and *The Year of Living Dangerously*, and author of the plays on which Bruce Beresford based *Don's Party* and *The Club*. 'Plays were cheaper than movies,' he explains, 'You could put on a play for $100 working with amateur actors. Even then movies cost at least $60 000 – they seemed totally impossible.' The impact of plays like *King O'Malley* can be understood in the light of Phillip Adams' recollection of trying to find actors for his first major film production. 'No one could do the accent,' he says, 'If you were an Australian actor you had to lose your accent almost immediately. Australians had played Tennessee Williams, Arthur Miller, Russian, French, Shakespeare, all sorts of plays, but unless they'd been in one of two stage plays in the fifties and sixties, they had never played an Australian!'

The introduction of televison to Australia in 1956 dealt a severe blow to cinema attendances. But paradoxically it meant as well a great advance for the possibility of a specifically Australian cinema: many of the people who would become involved in the film industry in the 1970s learned their craft in television, and acceptance by television audiences of Australian voices and stories paved the way for their acceptability in movies. The government ruling that commercials shown on Australian television should be produced in Australia meant that many people gained experience in camera, sound, design, and direction – and may help to explain a tendency towards glossy prettiness in many Australian films.

That many of the lobbyists for the reconstruction of a film industry were enthusiasts and writers on film also had quite profound effects on the character of the new Australian cinema. Through the sixties European films had become popular with a growing 'art house' audience, initially through the influence of the film festivals. The Melbourne Film Festival was organised by dedicated cineastes in the early fifties, and it had gained international respect, as had the Sydney Film Festival just a few years later. Influenced as well by the French critics of the New Wave era who made heroes of journeymen directors like John Ford, Samuel Fuller and Alfred Hitchcock, Australian critics were equally enamoured of Hollywood filmmaking. Still, their vision of an Australian national cinema was based principally on the models of the films being made in Sweden and France.

They wanted Australians not just to produce films, but to produce *good* films: notions of quality, integrity and reflectiveness were built into the very conception of what an Australian cinema should be like. And these qualities were directly linked with the issue of nationalism. Sylvia Lawson pointed out in an article for *Quadrant* magazine in

1965 that Ingmar Bergman's genius was embedded in his intuitive connection with Swedish landscape and culture; and that Bunuel's 'wrath and derision were formed in Spain, nourished in Mexico.' The cinema needed a nationalistic dimension, it was argued; but just as importantly, nationalism needed the cinema. A sense of national identity, wrote Lawson, is what 'a community's own filmmaking confers on it like nothing else.' Here was where the political arguments overlapped with the cultural ones. 'The film agitators ran a simplistic anti-American line,' recalls Phillip Adams, 'We said that we couldn't allow our children to grow up mimicking American accents, calling garbage cans "trash cans" and so on – even the colloquialisms were changing under the influence of American TV. The political argument was that we had to have a film industry so that we could stand on our own two feet.'

It was a persuasive argument in an Australia bubbling with the social, political and cultural ferment of the late sixties, and the politicians responded. First came the Experimental Film Fund, then in March 1970 the Australian Film Development Corporation. Soon after, an Interim Council for a Film and Television School to train people to work in the new industry was set up. Plans for the Film School almost foundered when John Gorton was displaced as Liberal Party leader and Prime Minister in 1971, but its fortunes, and those of the budding film industry as a whole, were soon revived. Expatriate Australians like directors Bruce Beresford and Ken Hannam began to come home. Beresford had left ten years before. 'At that time in Australia there was virtually nothing to do,' he says, 'When I was walking around saying I wanted to make films I was almost a lone voice. I thought the best thing to do was to go away to where people were interested – so I went to England.'

In 1972 the trickle of returning expatriates from all areas of the arts became a flood. In December 1972 a Labor government replaced the conservative Liberal-Country Party alliance which had ruled for 23 years. Their policies ranged from bringing home the troops from Vietnam, through restoring Australian resources to Australian ownership by trying to 'buy back the farm', to allocating even more substantial funds to the Australian Film Development Corporation. In 1975 the Corporation's role was expanded to include responsibility for both the Experimental Film Fund and Film

Australia, the government documentary production house which had been one of the few refuges for Australian filmmakers in the barren years of the fifties and sixties, when it was known as the Commonwealth Film Unit. The new body was renamed the Australian Film Commission. State governments too responded to the call – in 1972 the South Australian Film Corporation was established, and other states followed in the next few years.

The tone and style of the films that were made in the first seven or eight years reflected the nationalist orientation of the lobbyists. Two sorts of films dominated. The first stream were the 'ocker comedies', celebrations of that contemporary incarnation of the Australian larrikin, whose cheeky style, incompetence with or contempt for women and obsessive interest in beer had somehow come to define the popular image of the Australian. They included *The Adventures of Barry McKenzie* (1972), produced by Phillip Adams, directed by Bruce Beresford, and written by Barry Humphries, the Australian satirist who had created the quintessential ocker stereotype while an expatriate in London; and *Alvin Purple* (1973), about an ineffectual little man with a fatal attraction for women, produced and directed by Tim Burstall. The ocker comedies met with considerable popular success, supported by an audience who delighted in seeing people with their accents and their sense of humour walking around in their streets on a movie screen. The place of film stories had previously been an almost mythic territory: we were deeply familiar with the streets and sights of New York, London and San Francisco, but we knew them in the heightened way we knew the legendary lands of childhood stories. To see the everyday transformed and magnified on the screen, in the form of actor Graeme Blundell chatting up blonde TV personality Abigail on a Melbourne tram in *Alvin Purple* was both surprising and exhilarating.

But there were limitations to the ocker comedies. Director Gillian Armstrong points out that, 'The new middle-class cinema-going audience still regarded them as a bit cheap and nasty. I think *Picnic at Hanging Rock* was the film that first affected that audience. People felt, "We don't have to be embarrassed any more".' Peter Weir's 1975 lyrically gauzy film was beautiful to look at, celebrating the Australian bush and adolescent schoolgirls dressed in Victorian clothes, and its evocation of mystery was cinematically very powerful. Still, Bruce Beresford remains unrepentant about the criticism of the loutish Australian stereotypes in the ocker comedies. He maintains that Barry McKenzie was a harmless film and that anyway he was not working for some kind of national identity board.

Over the next five years the stream of Australian culture that desired refinement and gentility would be rewarded with a parade of 'period films', including Beresford's own *The Getting of Wisdom*. The Australian audience, for whom schoolroom history had meant largely British and European history and who knew more about the Wild West than about the settlement of Australia, devoured many of them voraciously. The training in image-making of the new film-makers had gained in television commercials bore fruit in the often superb photography and meticulous art direction. If there was a tendency to favour relatively bland stories with relatively innocuous characters, it didn't really matter to audiences. Nor were all the films of that kind: several of the films with a period flavour raised themes and issues which did more than flatter and soothe their audience, Phil Noyce's *Newsfront* (1978), Michael Thornhill's *Between Wars* (1974), and Ken Hannam's *Sunday Too Far Away* (1975), for example. The first of a string of widely acclaimed films produced by the South Australian Film Corporation, the achievement of *Sunday Too Far Away* was in its combination of a vivid evocation of the world of the shearing shed during the shearers' strike of 1956 with a serious examination of the tension between mateship and competition, through the character of Foley, the gun shearer, played by Jack Thompson.

The fact that the films themselves reflected the nationalist and 'quality film' aspirations of their original proponents is not too surprising. The public servants administering the funds shared these values, and were working within a charter framed by the government in precisely those terms. As well, several of the early lobbyists had themselves become producers of films – in Phillip Adams' words, many of those 'who got to make the films were those who had fought at the barricades'. The producer has a central position in the structure of the Australian film industry. There are no Australian film studios like the huge organisations which ran film production in the heyday of Hollywood, where writers, directors, cameramen and technicians were all salaried staff who worked when, where and on what they were told. And the government chose not to establish a state-run equivalent, like those in Czechoslovakia or Hungary, where technical and administrative support for film production were provided by a state authority. The Australian system, unlike any other, involved the allocation of funds to individual producers for production of particular films. Producers were also encouraged to raise finance from private sources: from the start the commercial viability of a project was a consideration of some importance. The ability of a national cinema to attract a paying audience for this genuinely popular art form was part of the rhetoric of the film lobbyists, and met a sympathetic hearing from governments presiding over the mixed Australian economy in which the prevailing assumptions are those of free enterprise. In John Gorton's 1970 speech he spoke not just of 'the improvement of the quality of life' which would follow from the establishment of a film industry: 'At least as importantly . . . as profit in human values . . . we expect profit in money terms.'

The 1972 election of the reforming Labor government did not automatically transform Australia into an independent filmmaker's paradise. One of the first actions by Doug McClelland, the new Minister responsible for the film industry, was to seek advice from Jack Valenti, the Executive Director of the Motion Picture Association of America. Coming at a time when there was a lot of discussion of the need to challenge the dominance of Hollywood movies in Australia's cinemas and the system of exhibition and distribution that had maintained it for so long, Valenti's visit met with less than enthusiasm from local filmmakers. When he arrived at a cocktail party in his honour at Sydney's Chevron Hotel he was greeted by 200 people with placards and slogans. They included many of the most famous and soon-to-be famous names in Australian film. The demonstration's high point was the dramatic appearance of a mafia boss and two floozies screeching to a halt at the Chevron's door in a black limousine, in a pointed entertainment directed by Peter Weir. Later in 1973 when a government-sponsored Tariff Board report recommended prohibiting exhibitors from controlling distribution companies and limiting the number of cinemas any one company could own, there was a flurry of protest from the exhibition/distribution section of the industry, Valenti was again consulted, and the provisions of the report were shelved.

It is producers in Australia who are in the crucial and powerful position of pulling a film project together. 'Australian producers have to have an extraordinary range of abilities,' says director Gillian Armstrong, 'they have to be entrepreneurs with the ability to con or enthuse businessmen into giving them money; they have to be able to pick projects that are going to work, and to pick the director and the team that will back the director; they have to be creative overseers of the project; and finally they are responsible for the marketing of it.' If producers had to answer to anyone in the early days it was to the government, the source of most of the funding. Over the first ten years of the new industry, an average of 50 to 60 per cent of a film's production costs, 75 to 80 per cent of marketing expenses, and 95 per cent of the vital script development funding came from the AFC.

One of the principal problems facing the new Australian films was in simply getting to an audience. Even in the 1970s the distributor/exhibitors were much more likely to buy an overseas film with a proven track record than an Australian film that was an unknown quantity in both the fact of its Australianness and in the ability of its director, actors and writer to deliver the goods in terms of audience response. In line with the emphasis in its charter on the need for some private support, and on the importance of reaching an audience, the AFC encouraged the distributors themselves to become involved in film investment, giving them a much greater interest in actually screening the final product.

The incorporation of distributors in decisions about which films would be made strengthened the Australian film industry's concern with commercial viability and with conventional assessments and assumptions about 'audience potential'. This direction for the Australian cinema was accelerated when in 1980 there was a change of tack, in the move to what the AFC's then Chief Executive Joe Skrzynski called 'Phase Two' of the Australian film industry. In keeping with the general economic policies of the post-1975 conservative government of Malcolm Fraser, which favoured reduction of all government expenditure, an attempt was made to shift the balance of funding for films from the public to the private sector through a system of tax concessions for film investment. In both the development of this system, and in the adjustments that have followed the first few years of its operation, the Australian film producers have played a significant role, just as they have in the development of particular films.

In general thinking, though, films are routinely presumed to be the products of their directors – we speak of 'Fred Schepisi's *The Chant of Jimmie Blacksmith*', and 'Peter Weir's *The Year of Living Dangerously*'. The pre-eminent director, enshrined in the 'auteur theory' which originated among the French critics of the sixties in the journal *Cahiers du Cinema* and was taken up by influential American critics like Andrew Sarris, has become part of conventional wisdom about film. Many directors are now as much celebrities as are the movie stars: the shutters clicked and bulbs flashed as wildly for Gillian Armstrong's entrance at the *Starstruck* premiere at Sydney's Hoyts cinema complex as they did for the arrival of the actors. Even so, the Star Director has not been a major feature of the Australian industry. The egalitarian style and the young-and-struggling nature of the industry demanded commitment and enthusiasm from all members of a film crew. The pressure to deliver quality results on very low resources meant that the Australian industry in its early days was a collective project, and it seemed that the interests of all involved coincided. But in recent times, this sense of co-operation has begun to show signs of erosion.

Since the move into 'Phase Two', the language of film producers must reflect the fact that the ears to which they address their pitch for money are no longer primarily those of public servants. Producers now have to orient themselves and their projects to the demands and assumptions of the accountants and lawyers who manage investment for the private sector, many of whom have little or no experience in film. The ability of a film to return the financial outlay of its backers has necessarily joined considerations like the aesthetic worth or the social value of a film at the very top of the priorities of those who make the decisions about which movies will be produced. At its worst, the tax legislation has allowed even commercial potential to become a non-issue: for some brokers film has simply replaced mineral exploration and macadamia farms as this year's model among legitimised tax-avoidance techniques.

Another crucial shift has been the increasing dependence of the Australian cinema on overseas sales: few Australian films with a budget of more than $500 000 can reasonably expect to recoup their costs on the home market alone. With Australia's small population, the enthusiasm of local audiences is simply not sufficient to generate net returns to producers and investors. The concern for overseas distribution of Australian movies has been part of the film industry's objectives from the very start, when it was argued that cinema was an effective way of raising Australia's international cultural profile. But in the early 1980s overseas sales became more than a good idea – they became an economic necessity. Sales to television networks in Europe and South America have long been part of Australian film producers' marketing strategies, but these outlets are small fry when compared with the returns promised by 'boffo box office', as the trade in America calls big attendances. Director Bruce Beresford points out, 'A population of fifteen million people back home is a ludicrously small audience for a movie. America is somewhere between 60 and 70 per cent of the world market for films, because it's such a wealthy society and there are so many outlets for movies, with television, cable and the huge numbers of cinemas.'

Reaching an American audience means in the first instance selling your film to an American distributor. Movies have been very big business in America for a very long time, and the lore that has grown up in Hollywood about what sorts of movies are likely to be successful, and for what reasons, is pervasive and powerful. Assumptions about the 'drawing power' of stars and about the sorts of stories audiences are judged to want, based on market research, previous successes and guesswork, underpin all decisions about what films a studio will invest in, and about what fully produced films will be bought for US distribution. Gillian Armstrong recalls taking her film *The Singer and the Dancer* around to American television networks and meeting with refusal after refusal. 'They'd all tell me that if next time I put in two American stars I might have more hope,' she says. While many Australian producers have so far resisted the temptation to make their films according to terms totally defined by the American movie business, it is clear that if US sales are sought, the conventional wisdoms of Hollywood filmmaking cannot be completely ignored.

Rising budgets – and the concomitant need for rising returns – and the government's move from a system of grants to a system of tax

concessions underlie a gradual shift in emphasis in the Australian
film industry. In parallel ways, and for some of the same reasons, the
collective spirit that characterised the Australian industry as a place
of work has changed since the early days. In 1979 a trend among
producers to bring in actors from overseas, particularly America, in
the hope of creating a more attractive 'package' for American buyers,
brought a strong reaction from one of the most influential film
industry unions, Actors' Equity. Uri Windt, then Assistant Federal
Secretary of Equity, explained that, 'We felt that the proposed use of
several imported artists in so many films put our interests, and the
very tone and nature of the film industry in jeopardy. There was a
spirit in the Australian industry that came from us all having fought
so hard to create it, but now we felt the producers were abandoning
the actors, so Equity said "no go". That led to quite a ruckus.' When
an attempt was made to import writers for films, the writers'
associations joined Equity in its opposition. And a move to bring in
overseas directors led to the formation of a Directors' Association in
1980 to defend the interests of directors.

Alongside the debate about the importing of overseas talent to
Australia is the debate about the reverse situation. Australian
directors are drawn to Hollywood by a variety of forces. Fred Schepisi
talks about the attraction of the 'pressure cooker' effect of working in
the biggest centre of filmmaking in the world. And most directors
share Bruce Beresford's views that recognition in America is
important to allow them to go on making films, and of Hollywood's
advantages of scale: bigger budgets and bigger salaries. Income from
his Australian films was very modest, says Beresford, and he had to
make commercials to supplement it. 'But in America the amount of
money you get paid to make a film relieves you of the burden of all
that.' For Peter Weir the question is not one of loyalty or betrayal of
his national origins. 'There are good films and there are indifferent
films,' he said on ABC radio at the time of the 1983 Cannes film
festival. 'With a good film the nationality is secondary. The film is its
own country.'

By the 1980s the quality and breadth of film themes and styles had
expanded dramatically, submerging the stream of ocker comedies
and period dramas. *Breaker Morant* (1980), directed by Bruce
Beresford was at one level a period film with a patriotic anti-British

thrust, but it also raised disquieting questions of the morality of soldiers in war. John Duigan's *Winter of our Dreams* (1981) developed a critique of the contemporary passivity of the many Australians who had been politically and intellectually active in the late sixties. *Stir* (1980), directed by Stephen Wallace, was a trenchant attack on the Australian prison system and its treatment of prisoners. Australian films were no longer predominantly comfortable and reassuring for their audiences.

And they were having far less trouble finding local distribution: it had been proved beyond doubt that Australian films could make money for the companies controlling distributors and cinema chains (though not always for their producers). In the summer of 1981-82, the films that drew the biggest audiences at Australian cinemas were *Mad Max 2,* (retitled *The Road Warrior* for its American release), the futuristic car-crash fable directed by George Miller, *Gallipoli*, director Peter Weir and writer David Williamson's vision of the historic massacre of Australian soldiers in World War One, and *Puberty Blues,* based on a book by two teenage girls about modern adolescence in a Sydney beach suburb. Directed by Bruce Beresford, *Puberty Blues* was produced by the successful team of Joan Long and Margaret Kelly. Then in 1982 came *The Man from Snowy River*, based on the Banjo Paterson poem about the triumphant ride of a young bushman. It became the highest grossing film ever in Australia. Produced by Geoff Burrowes and directed by George Miller (a different George Miller from the man responsible for the *Mad Max* films), *Snowy River* had beaten even all-time blockbuster record holders like the American *Star Wars* and *Gone With the Wind.*

Despite its diversity the Australian cinema does have a distinctive character. It rests partly on the look of the films, in how they are photographed, how the camera moves and the colour, lighting and composition of what it captures. The unique qualities of the Australian light and landscape also contribute. But as well there have remained some underlying themes that provide a certain coherence. There is a recurrent preoccupation with the bush and with the desert, although modern day Australia is one of the most highly urbanised countries in the world. The major characters in the films often have a self-effacing quality and sense of self-doubt that is a far cry from the heroes and heroines of classic Hollywood movie-making. At another level, many of the films choose to ignore the perspective – and often even the existence – of women, while others echo the incomprehension and embarrassment that characterised the ocker's relationship to sexuality in the early movies. The narratives of many of the films have an anecdotal, casual, almost documentary quality – there are not many grand adventures or epic exploits in Australian films. To all these general observations there are many exceptions – but the emergence of a distinctive Australian cinema is a phenomenon that has been remarked by critics and responded to by audiences in many parts of the world.

In the USA Australian films have enjoyed considerable success, although none have approached the sort of mass acceptance they have achieved at home. American critics and audiences have responded to what they perceive as the simplicity, innocence and directness of Australian films. According to New York *Daily News* critic Kathleen Carroll, 'There is a wonderful naive quality to the films, a freshness, a vigour. There is so much of that frontier spirit that we seem to have lost. They are reminiscent of our movies in the fifties and there is something comforting about that.' Other American critics have reacted against those qualities. For *New Yorker* critic Pauline Kael, 'There's no real excitement in them. "Australia" is almost like a Seal of Good Housekeeping on a movie. It's safe for a young man to take a girl to an Australian movie – a film that is terribly exciting can be upsetting to people out on a date . . . Australian films are like reading an old-fashioned novel.'

These perceptions are conditioned by the fairly limited range of Australian films which have been released in the US. The choice of which Australian films are shown in America is made by US distributors, but those decisions are influenced by which films are promoted most heavily at the Cannes film festival by the Australian government film bodies. Bruce Beresford's 1976 *Don's Party,* a critical vision of a beery Australian election party, was released in America only in 1982. 'I always knew it was talking about universal concerns,' says writer David Williamson. 'I remember the Department of Foreign Affairs doing everything they could to sink the cans of *Don's Party* at sea in transit, so that nobody outside Australia would ever get to see how badly we behaved.'

This embrace of Australian films by the American film business, critics and audience has pointed up a number of dilemmas for the Australian industry. Many have always been present as dormant tensions; others such as the attraction of some of Australia'a best film people to Hollywood (including several of the directors in this book) are completely new to the industry. The central question is how far the Australian industry should go in its dealings with Hollywood. Two opposing stances have developed. The first can be characterised as the internationalist approach, which favours accepting the assumptions and norms of the American industry and seeking universal appeal through employing American personnel in films which fit the patterns of mainstream Hollywood filmmaking. In the words of producer Tony Ginnane, one of the chief proponents of this view, 'In the real world of film exhibition and distribution where people actually go to the movies to be entertained, they don't care whether the films are made in Mongolia or Melbourne or Milwaukee.'

The other pole of the debate espouses 'cultural exactness'. In terms which recall the language of the film lobbyists of the sixties, they argue that Australian films have met with the success they have because of their direct connection with Australian society and culture. For screenwriter Bob Ellis, successful films 'have to tell what is commonly believed to be true. As the American director Mike Nicholls said, every film must ask you, "Does this remind you of anything, is this like your life at all?" If you can't answer yes, you won't go.' David Williamson concurs: 'While it's vital for the industry to make inroads into the American market, we shouldn't try to tailor our films for that. I think that path will lead to disaster.' To play too much by the rules determined in Hollywood they argue, is to risk the success of the films overseas and to jeopardise the values that led us to establish a film industry in the first place.

There is no easy resolution of this tension. Movies, like most forms of popular culture, are both commercial products and works of art. Filmmakers have to resolve often conflicting demands between what makes for good business and what makes for good art. Of all the people involved in the production of a film it is the director who finds her or himself at the heart of that contradiction. Just how and why that is so is one of the questions this book of interviews explores.

A movie is the final result of a multitude of decisions. It is a process involving politicians, financiers, producers, writers, cinematographers, camera operators, actors, composers and a vast array of people who perform technical tasks. It is the director's function, in George Miller's phrase, 'to ensure that everyone is on the same train'. In Fred Schepisi's words, 'to direct everything between the riverbanks.' Or as Gillian Armstrong puts it, 'Somebody has to filter all the information and keep a balance by saying yes or no. Finally it is the director's vision on the screen.' What makes up that vision, and what informs all those yes or no decisions are the questions at the base of these interviews with five of Australia's leading directors. The answers describe the evolution of the filmmakers' individual artistry; they also help illuminate the changing Australian culture that has determined the context, the material and the limitations of their achievements.

There are more than eighty directors listed in the *Australian Motion Picture Yearbook*. The five who were interviewed for this book are among the most widely known, and among the most successful. Their films range widely among the genres and styles that have emerged in the Australian cinema. In many areas their work style, their aesthetic style, and the way they understand what they are doing vary widely; on others they converge.

Like most of those who work in the new Australian cinema, all five directors in the book are relatively young. Their family origins reflect the diversity of contemporary Australia, from Fred Schepisi's Italian-Irish background, to George Miller's Greek origins, to the more traditional Anglo-Saxon ancestry of the others. All of them grew up in the affluence of the post-war period in Australia. As in many Western countries, the discovery by marketing men of the buying power of teenagers and the explosion in popular culture aimed at them through television, movies and especially rock and roll music, had given young people an unprecedented importance in the culture. Australia's prosperity afforded a rapid expansion in opportunities for tertiary education as the baby boom reached adolescence – as Fred Schepisi somewhat warily observed, four of these five directors have been to university or college. The optimism of the sixties, the sense Peter Weir described as 'the feeling that you could do anything, that everything would work out' was a powerful influence on many people's choices and it enabled many young Australians to ignore the conventional wisdoms about what was possible in Australia.

But there have been no easy rides for directors in Australia. The newness of the 'new' Australian film industry means that many of the difficulties faced by directors everywhere are magnified. The new Australian directors have had to discover and battle and master a multitude of problems without the backlog of acquired wisdom or the institutional supports that have evolved in older industries. Making films in Australia has demanded of all these directors an extraordinary level of commitment – 'you've got to be obsessed' is the way Fred Schepisi puts it. In this fledgling industry each director has had to recognise, understand and grapple with all three aspects of filmmaking stressed by George Miller when he describes movies as 'a business, an art, and a craft'.

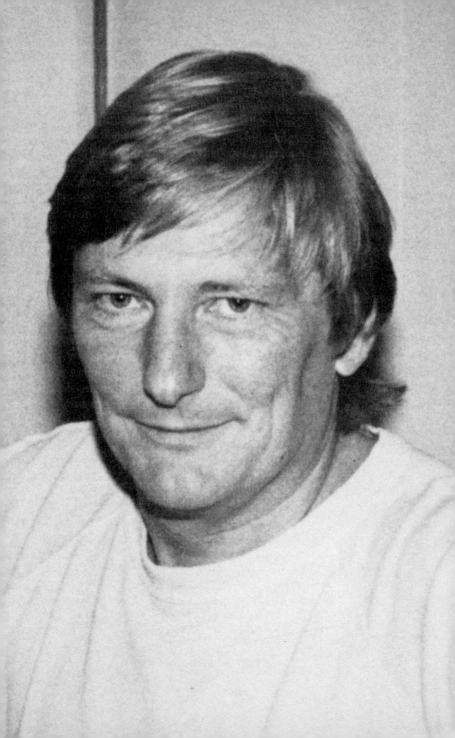

FRED SCHEPISI

Before this interview began Fred Schepisi asked who the other
directors in the book would be and wryly observed that he alone had
not been to university or college. This diffidence in Schepisi's manner
tempers the assurance of a self-confident Australian who has adopted
a few of the mannerisms of American business, where under-
statement is often viewed not as modesty but as stupidity. Dressed in
tan corduroy pants and a red sweatshirt with the words 'All
Australian Boy' on the back, Schepisi talked over two evenings in his
Los Angeles office after the day's work directing *Iceman.*

'Won't be a minute, love', Schepisi calls to the interviewer waiting
in his office. Sheets of plastic ice of differing colours and densities lie
around the room; scattered on the coffee table are polaroid snapshots
of potential Ice Men: casting is in progress and the key decision of
who is to play the rehabilitated Neanderthal must be made in the next
few days. On the walls are movie posters – one for *The Chant of
Jimmie Blacksmith,* Schepisi's 1978 film of the novel by Thomas
Keneally, one for Abel Gance's silent classic *Napoleon,* and one for
Barbarosa, Schepisi's first American film, made in 1982. As well,
there is an array of kids' drawings and many photos of Schepisi's six
children and present wife (he refers with a certain irony to 'my married
lives').

Fred Schepisi was one of the pioneers of the revival of Australian
cinema. His initial involvement in feature direction was *The Priest,*
one section of *Libido,* the 1973 feature made up of four stories, each
with a different writer and director. His first feature, *The Devil's
Playground* (1976), remains one of the finest Australian films. As
well as making films, Schepisi gave a lot of time to the activities of the
Producers' and Directors' Guild, to assessing student films at
Melbourne's Swinburne Institute of Technology, and to working on
the panel of the government sponsored Experimental Film Fund.

Director Gillian Armstrong notes how helpful Schepisi was to young
aspiring filmmakers in the early seventies, and how many Swinburne
graduates were given their first job at The Film House, Schepisi's
commercial production organisation. One of these graduates was Ian
Baker, the cameraman who has since collaborated with Schepisi on
all his films, even travelling to America to work with him on the Texas
shoot of *Barbarosa.*

Like many of those who made up the new cinema, Schepisi started
in television commercials. He credits film pioneer Phillip Adams with
having brought him into one of the major agencies; after that
Schepisi went into business for himself. Working in advertising
allowed him to develop business skills as well as filmmaking ones. He
built up his own production house, which gave him a base from which
to move into film direction and a group of technical people from which
to draw his crews.

It has been said that of all the new Australian film directors
Schepisi is the most successful cinema artist. His images have a rare
completeness. Like some of the European directors he admires, and in
a different way like the great Japanese ones, the composition and
lighting of shots in a Schepisi film are at once aesthetically pleasing
and entirely motivated by the sense and the substance of the film.

His films have received a mixed critical reaction. *The Devil's
Playground,* a semi-autobiographical story based on Schepisi's first
vocation, the priesthood, was set in a Catholic boys' seminary. It was
first shown at the Melbourne Film Festival in 1976 and met with a
very enthusiastic critical response. But Schepisi's next film, *The
Chant of Jimmie Blacksmith,* was flayed by the critics two years
later. Its graphic scenes of axe murder horrified a middle-class
audience accustomed to gentility and restraint in Australian films,
and its attack on the prejudice and hypocrisy of white nineteenth-
century Australians was probably a little hard to swallow after so
many period films had told us that really we'd been such very nice
people. *Jimmie Blacksmith* had its faults, but the savagery with
which it was dealt by the press was out of all proportion.

Soon after, Schepisi left for America. There the critical response, at
least, was more favourable. Pauline Kael in the *New Yorker* called
The Chant of Jimmie Blacksmith 'a masterwork', describing
Schepisi's direction as 'visually impassioned', adding, 'I don't think

there's an inexpressive frame of film in the entire movie.' Even so, as Schepisi explains, actually making films in Hollywood has proved far from easy.

Schepisi grew up in Melbourne, living first in Toorak, where his father had a fruit shop, then in Balwyn. 'My Dad had one of the first used car yards in Melbourne,' he says, 'before they became really bad.' He says he'd like to live between Australia and America. Home in Australia is now the Melbourne seaside suburb of Albert Park, close to the city and to The Film House. 'I like it there,' he says, 'I like the Victoriana, and being close to the beach. You can get on with working and then get back to your leisure as quickly as possible.'

Though he has acquired just a tinge of the West Coast in his accent, Schepisi's manner remains unmistakeably Australian – direct, informal and cheerful, he is an energetic man who gives the impression of not having much time for mucking about. He was the only director interviewed for this book who was not concerned to approve and amend the transcript. But if on the surface the purposefulness of the boy who insisted on studying to become a priest has been obscured by the easy assertiveness of the self-made man, you don't have to talk to Schepisi for very long to realise that it has not been entirely submerged. For all his larrikin air, Schepisi remains a serious and committed filmmaker.

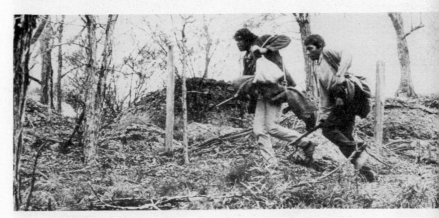

'I tried to construct every shot so you had to look for the Aboriginal in the frame before you found him, because he was so much a part of it.' Freddy Reynolds and Tommy Lewis in *The Chant of Jimmie Blacksmith*.

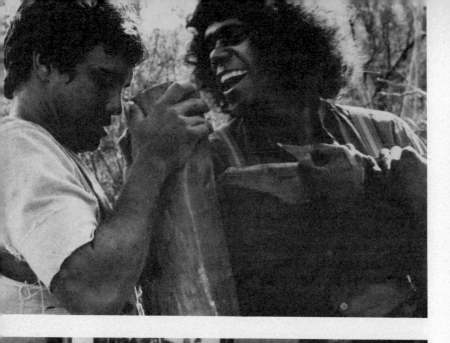

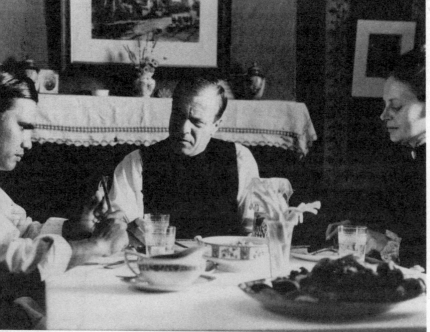

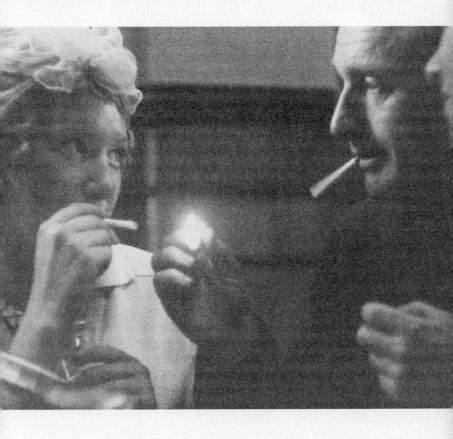

Above left: Tommy Lewis (Jimmie Blacksmith) and Freddy Reynolds (his half-brother Mort) fencing in *The Chant of Jimmie Blacksmith*.

Below left: 'Jimmie was pushed to the edge, split between black society and white society.' Tommy Lewis, Jack Thompson and Julie Dawson in *The Chant of Jimmie Blacksmith*.

Above: 'We gave ourselves a lot of agony using very fast lenses which mean you can light a match and have the light just explode on the actor's face.' Anne Phelan and Nick Tate in *The Devil's Playground*.

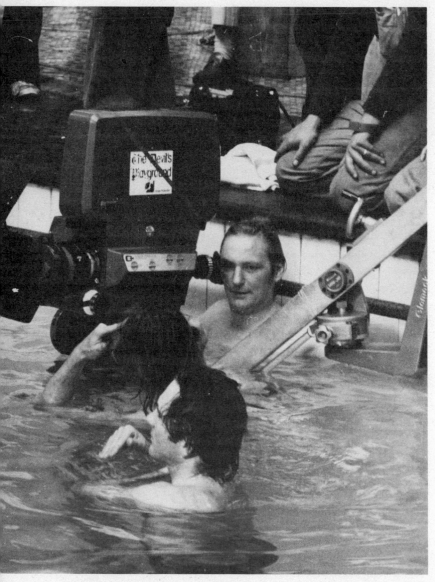

'The director is the one who directs everybody between the riverbanks.'
Fred Schepisi behind the camera on *The Devil's Playground*.

BEGINNINGS

Working Your Way Up

Sue Mathews: How did you come to pursue a career as a film director?

Fred Schepisi: When I was fifteen I decided I wanted to leave school – because I was impatient with it, not because I wasn't any good academically (as one writer reported, much to my annoyance). My parents didn't object because I was fairly headstrong and they knew if I didn't want to do it, I wouldn't. I worked with my father for a while in the car yards, but I was always very good at English and my mother thought we should find something for me to do – she always thought I was going to be a journalist. So when it was suggested to me that advertising was somewhere I could get paid very well for being good at English, I thought 'well, that sounds okay', being 15 years old and not knowing what the hell it was.

So I went to a vocational guidance test and the guy said 'what are you interested in' and I said 'I think I'm interested in advertising'. He said 'well, let's find out' and held up three cards: I got the colours right and he told me I was perfect for advertising. I got a job in an agency as a dispatch boy. I did that for a while until I convinced the company that they didn't need three dispatch boys and they'd be better off with a driver and a car. That fixed that. Fortunately we all got absorbed into other places in the agency and I went through press production, typesetting, and layout. I wanted to become an account executive because in those days account executives did everything, but at 16 they could hardly make me an account executive.

Fortunately television arrived in Australia and I got sidetracked into the television department. Most of the production companies were pretty raw at that time, so we were all experimenting together, both in writing and directing, though guessing was more what it was. At the same time I was getting very interested in 'Continental films', as we used to call them. They were so different from American and English films, not to mention hornier, which at fifteen or sixteen was fairly important. They seemed just extraordinary, they were so rich and involving. Clouzot's *Wages of Fear* with Yves Montand, and *One*

Summer of Happiness were the first two I remember, then Visconti's *Rocco and his Brothers,* and *The Fiends,* another Clouzot thriller.

How did you discover European films?
I think I went for entirely the wrong reasons. I went to see *One Summer of Happiness* because I thought I was going to see someone naked. It was the biggest disappointment of my life – I found out that the reason it was on the Catholic list was because it made fun of priests. But what I saw was a fantastic film and that piqued my interest from then on. I joined various film societies and I'd go to the Melbourne film festival. I went to see every different kind of picture I could, I fell in love with it.

I imagine in that early period in TV advertising you were able to get quite extensive experience.
I was very lucky from that point of view. I got to touch film, play with it, and get involved with the editing. We were always experimenting with techniques, trying to do something different. We would try to translate still-photography techniques, like bar relief, strange separation techniques, and high contrast things. And we'd try to come up with different ways to find a look without lighting – what struck me in French and Italian movies was how beautifully different the lighting was. Then filmmakers like Kurosawa began to influence the work I was doing with their use of exteriors and the way they used chemistry. I actually think we were the first people to use fog in commercials as a glamorous thing, to use weather textures and make them beautiful or exciting, to give energy, which is what Kurosawa does so incredibly well. As well, I was working with a number of art directors who helped influence the way I work now: in different styles, in patterns, on the square, and so on.

Are there any commercials of that period that you are particularly proud of?
Lipton jigglers was probably the most well known, I think, and we did a great many of the Marlboro commercials, with horses running through silvery water. And we were among the first people to use white limbo as a negative space, simply placing elements in it.

When did you move into your own production company?
When I was 24 I took a job as manager of Cinesound in Victoria. We made a profit within the first year, and by the end of the next year we were making more money than the parent company in Sydney. That was when I found out about loss companies. But it turned out to be for my benefit because, with my partners, I was able to buy the place.

Cinesound had been one of Australia's most productive feature film studios back in the thirties, then in the forties and fifties it was best known for its movie-theatre newsreels. Were the newsreels still important in your time?
We did newsreels, but when we bought the company I didn't take over the newsreels. I wasn't a very good newsreel person. I stopped my news crew going out when the Beatles came to Melbourne because I thought the mass hysteria was so ludicrous and dangerous that I didn't want to add to it. Another day, there was an aeroplane that had dropped an engine and was in big trouble. It was coming in to land and of course my news guys got all excited and were leaping into their car to go out. I thought it was incredibly ghoulish – it didn't seem to me to be reporting, just a desire to have a sensational piece of footage. So I took the keys and wouldn't let them go out. Newsreels were dying by then, anyway. There was only one person in the editing department when I arrived, an assistant editor called Russell Boyd who had been there for six months. Now, of course, he is one of Australia's foremost cameramen.

Where did you find the money to buy out Cinesound?
Three years before, when I was 22, I had borrowed £80 from a very sceptical bank manager to go up to Sydney with another guy to see Sir Norman Rydge, the head of Greater Union (one of Australia's three major exhibition-distribution chains), which all the way down the line owned Cinesound, Melbourne. I had a one and a half page report, and we made him an offer to let us take over the Melbourne end of Cinesound for no money and eventually pay it back. To my amazement he actually listened to us for about three quarters of an hour. Of course we didn't convince him to hand over Cinesound, but subsequently I got the job of managing it. After two years I went back to him and said 'you remember me, I've been running your company

and you can see what I've done. So let me put it to you this way, why don't we do it on the terms I suggested before.' He agreed and I bought Cinesound for almost nonexistent money down, with a promise to pay back specific large lumps over a couple of years. He seemed impressed that I'd tricked my way into the joint and made money, so he let me have it. That's how my company, The Film House, started. I thought I was going to make movies straight away.

Was that the motivating force from the age of 16?
Well I thought I liked advertising when I was 16, but I lost that urge very quickly, I just didn't like the business at all. The idea was to make money to make films, but then there's the reality of what films cost. Also you get involved in a business and suddenly you're involved in it fifteen hours a day. You're as busy as you can possibly be and you are expanding and getting equipment and maybe doing a lot of turnover, but you've got to keep churning the money back to improve the facilities. You find yourself on this amazing wheel where you seem to have a lot of money, but if you get off the wheel you lose it all. So I got caught up in business in a big way, in a nightmarish way. I didn't have holidays, I managed the place, I wrote most of the commercials, I wrote the documentaries, and I directed them.

The Revival Begins in Melbourne

Was anybody making feature films at that time?
There was the odd film here and there. Tim Burstall was doing a lot of the spadework, he was the original battering ram. At that time he was doing *2000 Weeks,* a feature which was a lot better than people gave it credit for, and not long after, I think, he made *Stork.*

Was there a circle of people interested in filmmaking in Melbourne at that time?
Tim Burstall was part of a group that was based in the outer suburb of Eltham, an art colony that had been established for a long time. They were into every form of the arts and Tim led them into film. They really put everything into it, with no money, no help, no backing. They

made a lot of pioneering inroads. Then there was the Carlton push which was a later development, a younger group that came out of universities and technical colleges. And then there was the professional ring, the would-be filmmakers working in related areas such as the ABC, who really weren't doing anything.

Burstall was a key person in the Producers' and Directors' Guild and I got involved in it because I hoped I'd meet a lot of theatre people. I wanted to learn about play structures and dealing with actors and performances and how theatre was different from film. The Producers' and Directors' Guild turned into quite a catalyst: we all fired one another up and began trying to generate things for television, film, and stage. We recognised a need for unity and help. We would run competitions for scripts and produce them on stage, on film and on television.

You did all this in your spare time?
Yes. At the same time I was involved in the Experimental Film Fund as one of the assessors, sometimes referred to as one of the assassins. We used to deliberate for hours over hundreds of scripts. We used to take every one at face value, trying to think from the writer's point of view, and trying not to do any smart dismissals. In most cases we were only talking about $300, but that amount was so precious we really had to take it seriously. The Experimental Film Fund did a remarkable job – it got *Stork* off the ground, and gave people some basic opportunities to experiment or prove themselves.

Was the activity in Melbourne very different from what was going on in Sydney at that time?
The Experimental Film Fund was going in Sydney as well. The film course at Swinburne technical college was already going in Melbourne, quite some time before the national Film and Television School started in Sydney. The attitude to making movies in Sydney was much more Hollywood. They wanted job demarcation, unionisation, more glamour, and more money. In Melbourne we used smaller crews, there was more cross-pollination of jobs, with everybody working to one end. We were closer to the Czechoslovakian or Swedish approach. Even among the competitive commercial companies in Melbourne, we would all help one another.

If someone had a problem they would ring up, and if we could solve it for the other person, even though we had just lost the job to them, we'd do it. I think that had a lot to do with us actually getting things off the ground.

MAKING   THE   MOVIES

Libido

Your first involvement with a feature film was The Priest, *the episode you directed of the four-part Libido in 1973. How did you come to be involved with the project?*
Through the Producers' and Directors' Guild we had been encouraging people from other media to write for film, television and stage. We asked people to submit scripts on the theme of libido, and we produced the film ourselves. I knew Thomas Keneally, the novelist, was submitting a script. At that time I was planning on writing *The Devil's Playground* but I didn't know whether I was capable of it, so I thought maybe I should get to know Tom Keneally, just in case I got into trouble. The other thing that attracted me to Keneally's story of the nun and the priest was that I thought directing two people in one room for half an hour was probably the most difficult thing I could handle at that time. So I went right for it – I didn't give anybody else a chance at that one. And while we were discussing *The Priest*, Tom Keneally had *The Chant of Jimmie Blacksmith* in galley proofs and it was then that I started my campaign to get that. It took me a few years to get it off him.

It's interesting that your first two feature productions have to do with sexual repression and the Catholic church.
Well that's coincidental because of the rather arbitrary way I selected *The Priest*. On the other hand I was passionate about *The Devil's Playground*. But I liked both subjects and I'm glad I did them. My ex-wife Rhonda did the casting for *Libido* and we had two fine theatre actors, Arthur Dignam and Robyn Nevin. They had never acted in a film before, and so were very interested in the process. They were a

great help to me and vice versa. I wanted to work everything up out of the camera, a bit too much I think, and I had worked out a very definite camera structure to enhance the drama. I thought the script was overwritten, and we took out a lot of words in rehearsal, a lot in shooting, a lot in editing, and we could probably have taken out more. It was a terrific experience; two actors and a crew who really cared, and Gillian Armstrong who was a student in the film course at Swinburne, was doing the tea.

The Devil's Playground

How long after that did The Devil's Playground *get under way?*
I think it was 1971 that we worked on *Libido*. It took me until 1975 to get to do *Devil's Playground*.

Were you working on the screenplay during that time?
I had done the screenplay shortly after *Libido* and it took me two and a half years to raise the money. In fact most of that was me earning it. The Film Commission initially would not give me any money: I applied to them again and again and again. But even though they weren't enthusiastic, nobody in Australia had won as many awards as I had in both documentaries and commercials, so eventually I got about $100 000 worth of acknowledgement. I put $154 000 in and I raised the rest in lots of $1000 and made the film. When I finished it nobody liked it or wanted to distribute it, so I had to raise the money to distribute it myself. It meant that I came off that film exhilarated, but I had to go straight back to work doing commercials. I would work during the day and do a second lot of work at night. The film was being edited at the same time. It was not the happiest period of my life. It was very tough, but I insisted that it was a commercial picture and made sure that it was treated that way.

You had been thinking since 1971 of doing that film. How long had the idea of doing an autobiographical film about that period of your adolescence been an ambition?
I was reading a lot of books looking for a subject, and around 1971 it just crossed my mind that it might be an interesting world to explore

as a film. I made notes for nine months: plots, thoughts, pieces of action, and possible endings and middles. I wrote lots of ideas in a book and then somebody stole it. It was horrendous for me as well as being vindictive.

You think it was a deliberate sabotage?
Yes, I fired somebody around the same time. So I couldn't face it for a long time. Some time later, I was writing a documentary for Film Australia – I used to shoot commercials and run the business during the day, then write at night. One night I finished more quickly than I expected and went to bed four hours early. Then *The Devil's Playground* started coming, so I got up and started writing. It took me about two months. I used to work every morning until three or four in the morning and then get up and go to work. I'm not sure I could do that any more.

To what extent did you draw on your own experiences? How much of you is there in the character of the boy, Tom?
It's semi-autobiographical. When I was thirteen I decided I wanted to enter the monastery, and I think my parents made the wisest decision and let me do it. I left a year and a half later, by which time had got it out of my system. The Brothers are combinations of various people; the events are combinations of what happened to me and to other people and some of them are made up. Once when I was about nine I was in the infirmary of my Catholic primary school, which happened to be right next to the Brothers' billiard room, so I could hear some of the conversations, and once I stayed back for a few days at the end of term; they were more relaxed under those circumstances, so I briefly got inside their world. The film was really made up of what I thought it would be like, and what I thought was going on, or, if you like, extensions of what I thought I might have become.

You would see yourself presumably as closest to the Nick Tate character who is the most approachable, and the most confused, of the Brothers.
I hope so. I'm sure I wasn't that far away from the Arthur Dignam character either. No, I hope I'd never let that beast out.

How do you feel about that period of your life? Do you feel any anger or resentment?

No I don't, it's just what I went through. I think a lot of it is very silly, and I'm definitely against it, but, no, I don't feel any bitterness about it. I don't think that those people were doing that to me deliberately or with malevolence: they thought they were doing the right thing.

There's a point where the Nick Tate character is reflecting on how he feels about life in the seminary and he says apparently without irony, 'I love all this brotherhood, I feel I belong here.' I was wondering how you intended that?

I believe that. He didn't agree with it all, and quite clearly hadn't come to terms with a lot of it, but he liked the life, and that's a fact, they do. I wasn't trying to paint the Brothers as black. They are products of a system and were trying to do the best they could, believing they were doing the right thing while maybe doubting some things. They taught obedience which is one of the vows, so it's pretty tough.

The Arthur Dignam character is very bitter and repressed, with his punishments of the boys and guilt-ridden visits to the public baths to watch women undressing. It's a very extreme characterisation.

That's what you think. I don't care what anybody says, I backpeddled a long way on how extreme I made that film, mostly because I didn't think people would accept it if I gave them any more, but the eccentricities of the people in that environment are a lot less than they really were. I can tell you that the Arthur Dignam character is a mere shadow of a couple of the people I experienced. When the film came out, people used to ring me up and write me letters and burn their T-shirts and send them to me. Almost any Catholic boy who has been to boarding school will say of that character 'that was Brother —.' There was one in every school, and they'd say to me 'oh, you were kind to him.'

How similar to Tom's was your experience of deciding to leave?

I did run away once but really it was quite different. I got to the point where I thought 'this life's not for me', because I liked girls a lot. Though like Tom I used to wet the bed a lot and the part where he is given the Lourdes water to cure his bedwetting is true – I made a small deal with myself that if the Lourdes water didn't work in one month I was going to give it up. It didn't work. So I told them I wanted to leave and they actually did pull me out of class one day when least expected, saying 'get your pen and leave' and drove me home. They were quite nice about it, though not being able to say goodbye was very strange. I never wet the bed again.

That was your first feature. Were there many lessons that you learned or surprises about the way it turned out?
Sure, but I can't tell you what they were. I think the saddest thing was that I didn't have the opportunity to immediately go on and apply the lessons that I had learnt, the economies of doing things. I actually learnt more out of seeing it recently than I did at the time.

What sort of things?
There are some things, like how cold the water in the showers is, that are repeated so often I thought 'if you say that again I'm going to tear the screen down.' Probably because I did some of the cutting myself there are some set-ups missing, and some things seem to come in right out of the blue so that you think 'where the hell did that come from, it has no relevance to anything.' And the writing was a little overwrought in places, a little too clever. Amazingly though, an incredible energy and honesty comes through which overrides and excuses all of it. It doesn't excuse it for me but it does for the audience. But it's very raw. I've come a long way since then.

The director of photography, Ian Baker, came to Filmhouse from the Swinburne film course, and he's worked on all your features so far. How closely together did you work on deciding how something was going to look?
I like to work up my action out of the camera, so we work very closely. We discussed everything, kept pushing one another away from the camera. We do it very co-operatively, because each composition is affected by a range of things. For example, by the sound I'm using off

screen, because that's giving information I don't need to put on screen; or by the approach I'm using in design and cutting. Composition adds an emotional impact as well. We discuss the lighting then Ian does it, but we do the composition together because it affects the cutting, not just a specific shot. As years have gone on we speak less and less because we know what we're doing and why we are doing it.

There are some terrific shots in The Devil's Playground, *like the repeated shot of Tom running down the stairs where you are looking almost through the floor.*
One of the reasons we picked that particular location was because the stairwell was open at one end, so we were able to do that. It's a crane shot and what makes it work is the lighting – that's why you need real co-operation with your director of photography.

I like the opening too, where the camera slowly tracks along the river to where a group of boys are diving and playing.
Yes, we were hanging off the front of a boat. That water is so shallow you wouldn't believe it – when they dive bombed they hit the bottom. It was also freezing cold. We wrote the film to be shot in a number of seasons and planned to do certain things in autumn and into winter. But in fact the lake shot was screwed up – we had a camera shaft break on us without us knowing and we lost the first – and hottest – day's shooting, so we had to come back and do it on a very cold day, much to everybody's delight.

Another shot I liked very much comes towards the end, where Tom and the old Brother, Sebastian, are talking on a balcony. They are framed above the line of stone columns.
That was originally going to be done in the sun – I thought I'd like to repeat the opening, where Tom first sees Sebastian sitting in the sun. We only had that particular actor for three weeks and we scheduled the scene five different times, and each time the weather just blotted us out. So in the end I had to come up with an entirely different concept, had to say 'where can I shoot this thing where it's kind of outside and isolated and away from other people but protected from the rain?' Answer – the balcony. And it makes it doesn't it? You know,

somebody else makes movies, you just have to follow it. Providing
you know why you are making the film or what your discipline is, you
can make those adjustments, but boy, somebody else makes the film;
obstacles just appear in your path so there's only one way you can go.
It's like going down a river, where as long as you stay within the
banks, you're okay.

*How was it working with the young boys? Were they professional
actors?*
No, not really, though the lead actor Simon Burke has gone on to an
acting career. We spent a lot of time in rehearsal and training and
everybody was given a very definite character and biography, a
nickname and an attitude to other people. If you get the right kids,
you find they really like acting. If you can tap that and lose the
embarrassment, you've got it made, and we really had terrific kids. As
in all my Australian films Rhonda Schepisi put an extraordinary
amount of work into selecting the cast.

*A lot of the subject matter deals with issues like masturbation
that must be difficult for kids – for anyone – to deal with in public
in that way.*
It was handled very carefully and I tried to grade the shooting to lead
up to that, and I kept talking about it so by the time it arrived it was
almost anything to get over it with. When the time came it was 'come
on, we've got ten minutes, we've got to be out of here, we haven't got
any time for this messing around, get on with it.' So there was no
choice. I used every trick a director has for getting something out of
somebody, from coercing, to taking breaks, to lecturing, to getting
tough, to getting nice.

*The final shot is of Tom in the car. He realises that he's got away –
it's a lovely expression on his face – and then the focus shifts to
the reflections of the trees and the sky on the car window going
past. Had you decided from the start that you were going to end it
like that?*
Oh yes, heaven and earth, definitely. We shot that on the first day – I
figured no easy introductions, let's get the kid off the ground in a big
way.

The Chant of Jimmie Blacksmith

You mentioned working with the writer Thomas Keneally as early as Libido *in 1973, and you gave him a small part in* The Devil's Playground, *as the priest who preaches on the horrors of hell and gives Tom Lourdes water for his bedwetting. He also appears briefly as a shearer's cook who might possibly be the father of Jimmie's child in* The Chant of Jimmie Blacksmith. *How closely did you work with him on the adaptation of the novel? First of all, how did you manage to extract the rights to the book from him?*

It wasn't until after I'd done *Devil's Playground*. There were quite a few people in various places in the world trying to get the rights. Tom really wanted to sell it internationally – at that time there was nothing much happening in the film industry in Australia. But I think he liked what I'd done with my films and I was able to offer him cash, split across a couple of financial years, and that's what finally swung the deal: he wasn't terribly wealthy at the time.

He'd written the novel during what he considered a black period of his life and he didn't quite like some of the attitudes of the book, so in fact I wrote the screenplay on my own. I showed it to him when I finished and I remember he kept rushing to the book to find out whether the good bits were his or mine. They were mostly his. I really did try to encourage him to get involved, but he didn't want to at that time. He was taken aback by the power of the thing and I think he was very worried that it was going to unleash some kind of riot. The imagery was so violent and strong on film and maybe it made him feel rather strange about what he had written.

How did you go about the process of adaptation? How closely did you refer to the novel as you were writing the screenplay?

I broke the book down on a series of little cards and stuck them on the wall. Then I wrote two movies in structure form, using the cards. I wrote the movie I made, and I wrote a movie that started with the school teacher being kidnapped, which comes at the end of the story chronologically. The time of the movie was the whole time they had him kidnapped. I did it that way because I was interested in doing it in flashbacks. The school teacher would be wrangling with the kidnappers, so that you would be instantly involved in action and threat. Under that tension the audience, like the school teacher, would be trying to learn who these threatening characters were. The teacher and the audience know they've been killing people and you'd flash back to pieces of what they'd done so that in a way you'd prepare the audience for the horror so that by the time you unleashed it, the audience would be both prepared for it and would understand why it happened. I'm not convinced that that may not have made the film a lot more commercial, but I liked the way we went anyway.

Had the theme of the movie been important to you for a long time? What was it attracted you to the book in the first place?
The story of a man at odds with the system who just wants to be himself and get on in the system. That's probably what attracts me to most material.

The story is about a young part-Aboriginal who has been brought up by a white missionary in the nineteenth century. He tries to find work and establish a life for himself in the first part of the film. Had the treatment of the Australian Aborigines been an issue of particular importance to you?
A cause celebre? Not particularly. It had always disgusted me, but I wasn't actually doing anything about it. The story caught me, it seemed to me to be a very entertaining way to explore the plight of the Aborigine, and it had such imagery in it. A number of elements attracted me to it. It was never meant to be the definitive Aboriginal picture, as everybody seemed to expect, because that's just not possible. They are more complex than we are and there are more diverse groups or tribes.

How did you research it? I find it easier to imagine how you'd familiarise yourself with the classic stuff of anthropological research than with the shanty town scenes. Where did you develop your ideas of how they should look and what they should feel like?
From seeing films from the past. From being in places like that, in the Northern Territory and around Alice Springs, and by doing research. You've got to give Wendy Dixon and the art department

an enormous amount of credit. They did a lot of research and a lot of incredibly clever work. The design on that picture is quite phenomenal, right down to the one thing that probably nobody knows – the book that the school teacher kept wanting to take with him. 'My Palgrave,' he kept saying, 'I want to take my Palgrave.' What the hell is that? Is it boots, or a scarf? It's a little book of poetry which Wendy had on a shelf, annotated in the character of that school teacher, so that when the actor walked on the set and was looking around, he discovered the Palgrave and it just heightened the performance. Wendy's design was beyond something that you see as an audience, it created an atmosphere and ambiance for the actors which I think is just incredible. In fact, everyone's contribution on that film was extraordinary. It always tends to come out as 'the director did it all', which is nonsense. The sound is terrific; and a lot of credit must go to Roy Stevens, who was production manager, because he made me contain the picture. We had to cancel locations and come up with new locations and he made us go that extra ten per cent, take that extra time, but cut that corner whenever possible.

Had you seen many of the other films that had been made in Australia about Aborigines?
To tell you the truth, I thought most films made about Aborigines were wrong. They seemed superficial: they always had them with the spear and the leg up on the knee, standing on the horizon. I don't think Aborigines would be that silly. They were part of the earth, they were in harmony with it, they lived with it, so I tried to construct every shot so that you had to look for the Aboriginal in the frame before you found him, because he was so much a part of it. He was always shot down into the earth, against a hill, in amongst the trees, so that he never stuck out on the horizon. He was always part of it, in harmony with it, whereas the white person stuck up out of the earth, he was at odds with it, taking from it.

You use a lot of close-ups of insects, textures of bits of wood and bark and so on.
It's a discipline of the film. The Aboriginals perceived the bush as alive with food, insects, nature to cohabit with, where we tend to see nothing. Sometimes those shots represented the passing of time,

sometimes they were a comment on the action, sometimes they were just showing what was in the environment.

You also emphasise the chooks that seem to be on all the White farms.
Well they were the animals that were being used then. And there was the suggestion of violence, with the farmers chopping the heads off and hanging them up. I was trying to say that the whites were used to killing, more than we are today. They were used to violence, it was part of the way they lived and ate.

Where did you find the Aboriginal actors?
We had searched through black theatre in Sydney, where we did find a lot of our actors, and we searched all up the coast of NSW. We found Tommy Lewis, who plays Jimmie, in an airport. My wife and I were fog-bound in an airport. I noticed him and then Rhonda noticed him and we talked it over and she chased after him and chatted him up. We tested him over about four days. Tommy was a student at the time and we went to a break-up party for his course where a couple of other blacks came along. One of them was Freddy Reynolds, and the minute he walked through the door, I said 'that's Mort'. He was just right.

What have Tommy Lewis and Freddy Reynolds done in the time since making that film?
Freddy has not done very much unfortunately. The last I heard, he was lecturing at schools. It's difficult, people didn't exactly rush them with roles, though I don't know why. It took a long time for people to understand how good Tommy was, they somehow thought it was me and Michael Caulfield, the acting tutor on the film, doing it. But you can't put a cinemascope camera right in on the eyes of a person and have that subtlety of emotional change register unless it's coming from within the person, unless he is doing it. Now, of course he is getting work in TV and films which is terrific.

It must be a very difficult adjustment to make, for people who've never been performers.
That's true for anybody who gets into that limelight. I was very

careful, as I was with Simon in *The Devil's Playground,* to say 'this is an event, this is a holiday, it may never happen again. When it's over, remember the holiday, it was great, but don't chase it for the rest of your life.' But when you've got somebody like Tommy who is in every scene and you don't want him to move, you deliver him things – a cigarette, a drink, you wipe his brow – and then it's not very long before he's demanding: 'cigarette!' The first time you hear that you've got to stop them, admonish them, send them off the set for arrogant behaviour, get them back to earth again. Then there's the publicity tour afterwards, and the girls. Those guys pull birds like you've never seen in your life and it's a big high.

It's a real responsibility, getting someone who's not an actor, who's not prepared for it, into that sort of experience.
Yes, definitely. And the pressures aren't just from this side of the fence, they are also from their own people. Take someone like Freddy who's been really screwed by the system, a fullblood Aboriginal with no tribal heritage whatsoever, taken away from his parents at a very early age and shoved in some white boarding house somewhere. He's been at war with the whites since he was five, and then we take him and dote on him. The strain on anybody fresh walking into a movie is extraordinary and the strains on somebody like that are beyond the pale, I'm afraid. And with Tommy, while on the one hand he liked to be in the city, he couldn't be there very long because he really was a person who would go out hunting, and he liked that. I think he's found a reasonable balance in both worlds. Finding a balance between ordinary life and the life when you're in a movie is hard for all actors – both worlds don't keep going constantly: even Jack Thompson is out of work for long periods of time. So we tried to keep setting precedents as the picture went on. But at the same time, you make a movie, you increase your family in a lot of cases. It's a very intimate and enjoyable experience and you are never totally separate from then on.

At the time it was the biggest budget film that had been made in Australia wasn't it?
'Death of the Australian film industry,' they said, 'the biggest, most

disgusting budget ever.' Why did I want to make a big budget film? I
wanted to make *The Chant of Jimmie Blacksmith* and I wanted to
make it on the scale that it should have been made and there wasn't
one penny spent needlessly. Today, executive producers are ripping
off $200 000 and more for putting the package together. For writing,
producing and directing *The Chant of Jimmie Blacksmith* I got
$36 000, plus I paid cash for the rights. I didn't even get paid in the
end, but that was what I was written down for. And I invested
$250 000 in the film. Everybody got stuck with rotten money and it
was done in the most economical way possible. It just happened to
cost that much.

*There was a big publicity build-up at the time it was released and
while it was being made. Was that a conscious marketing
decision?*
Yes, of course, but there was one major problem. We achieved
something that nobody else had achieved, in getting into the Cannes
film festival international competition. Given the politics of the Cannes
festival, and how prizes are awarded, to be the first of the new crop of
Australian films ever to get into that festival was an end unto itself, it
was the award. The problem was that suddenly everybody was
predicting we were going to win awards. That's when I thought the
publicity had gone crazy. I tried to stop it, but how do you stop it? When
I came back, the customs officer said 'gee, sorry about you failing
overseas.' We didn't fail, we got a five-minute standing ovation.

How did that feel?
Extraordinary. I always get embarrassed with that stuff, so I think the
people who were with me, my father-in-law and brothers-in-law, got
more of the feeling that I would have liked to have got out of it.

*Was the Cannes screening before or after the film's Australian
release?*
Before. I'd walk down the street in Melbourne and someone would say
'sorry about your film, buddy.' And then, everybody expected it to be
definitive, they expected every dream they ever had of an Aboriginal
picture to be in it, and they certainly didn't expect it to hit them across
the head.

How do you feel now about the graphic violence in the film?
It was necessary, you can't not have it. The film is making a very
definite anti-violent statement. It's not glamorous, it's not romantic
and it certainly didn't sell tickets, but it's necessary. The point is that
violence happens when you least expect it, to the people that you least
expect or want it to happen to, and it is committed by a person who
you don't want to do it. It's sickening and vile and all it does is beget
violence.

*Did you expect the character of Jimmie Blacksmith to retain the
audience's sympathy?*
I clearly expected to lose it the minute he killed. I expected to get it
back through the affability of the brother, Mort. The intention was to
use Mort to bring the audience back around to Jimmie again. I don't
know whether I did that for you – did I?

Well, no, not really.
It's fifty-fifty: with a lot of people I did and a lot of people I didn't.
Some people are drawn right into the film from the beginning and
have no trouble with what's happened to Jimmie or why. But the same
element that sucks people in seems to push others right outside the
film – there's no middle ground.

*Part of the reaction against the film may be a sense that you don't
judge Jimmie, that you let him off too easily.*
He gets the shit beaten out of him. He's not let off by the people. I do
not say that he is guilty; I say he was pushed to the edge, split between
black society and white society. He is not a black, he is a half-caste and
he can't belong to either society. So in the end it is just inevitable to
strike out. It isn't what he should have done, but what the hell else
was he going to do.

*There are a lot of other things besides picking up an axe and
chopping people up.*
Maybe it was the white component that made him take up the axe, and
not the black component, maybe it was forces beyond his control. He
struck at women, because of tribal things against women, and
because it was women whose love he most desired but couldn't get. It
was an act of frustration, a moment of frenzy without really realising

what he was doing. But why try to make a judgement of it? It's a fact,
like many criminal acts, and the film is an examination of what
brought it about.

What sort of models did you have of how to present the violence?
Was Sam Peckinpah an influence at all?
No, definitely not. There was very little blood in the film. In fact I tried
to develop something that would attenuate the experience of death,
the horror and the pain of it, by going unexpectedly to people's faces,
maybe to a face you didn't expect, then onto the face you did expect,
but with an unexpected reaction. There is very little actual violence,
but somehow the experience is worse than if there was more.

Did you re-edit the film for its overseas release?
Yes, the version of *Jimmie Blacksmith* that was released overseas
was much better. There is about twelve minutes missing, mostly after
the killings. I decided that once those killings had happened, you
really owed it to the audience to wrap it up and let them out of the
theatre to get a breath of air. What I was doing in the original version
was going on and exploring what was happening to the country,
people's reactions, and other reasons for it happening. I now realise –
and this is something I learned even more on *Barbarosa* – that there's
a certain point beyond which you mustn't introduce any new
information that requires you to go off and think in a new direction.
There's an emotional drive that you have to follow and allow to be
concluded, and any new information must pertain only to that –
otherwise you dissipate the energies of the film. It's not a novel, it's a
film: it's a physical experience as much as anything else, and you've
got to let that drive take you through.

B a r b a r o s a

Why did you make Barbarosa? *From reading the account that you*
gave in the Playboy *interview, it sounds like it was almost*
'because it was there'.
It was almost that, except that I wouldn't do anything like that. You
have to make your first American film, and until you have made an

American film, no matter what you've done anywhere else, you don't have any credibility here. Their reasoning is that the conditions in Hollywood are different, but their real reasoning is that nothing else matters. *Barbarosa* had the country singer Willie Nelson, who's a persona; it had Gary Busey, who I believe to be a terrific actor. The story was interesting. I hadn't intended, though, to do another picture in the country, in the outback, and I did not want to do another picture with basically men. I wanted to be in a studio full of women. Not really, but I wanted to do something different.

It had some interesting themes in it, about people needing people, about families staying together and being a unit. There's a strange little theme in there about hatred as a uniting force, which was worth examining. Beyond that it was a romp with two guys, a bit like *Butch Cassidy and the Sundance Kid,* but with a little weirdness about it. I did it as an entertaining adventure picture.

The family seems to be a central theme in your films. It's there in Barbarosa *too: it's the story of an outlaw played by Willie Nelson, who has been thrown out of his Mexican wife's village by his father-in-law. The rest of his life seems to be spent circling round the campesino in a constant feuding balance, so that his wife's family remains the centre of his existence.*
That interested me as one of the subthemes in what I saw as entertainment. But it was a large part of what interested Bill Witliffe, the writer, and I thought I'd like to achieve that in the film.

On the credits I noticed it's a Witliffe–Nelson–Busey production. What did it actually mean, to have your writer and your two stars as your bosses?
A headache. They packaged it, they put the project together. In actual shooting it meant that Bill Witliffe got involved, Gary Busey tried to get involved, and Willie, well he didn't care in terms of producing. Then there was another producer, plus the executive producer of the company. Mostly I tried to realise what Bill Witliffe wanted, because he was the one who wrote the script and it had been his passion for many years. We had some differences over things in the script – things I thought might interrupt the compelling energy that emerged between the two main characters – but I was not trying

to make Fred Schepisi's film, I was trying to realise Bill Witliffe's film.

Have you always been interested in westerns?
No, not particularly, though I do like some of the great westerns. I certainly didn't come here to do a western. It was an interesting challenge, because it's a very different kind of western and yet I wanted to deliver certain elements of the genre. Ian Baker and I looked at some old westerns, observing costuming, and what might or might not have been valid, but a lot of the time we were looking at clichés to avoid.

Do you feel as satisfied with the use of the landscape in Barbarosa *as in* Jimmie Blacksmith?
Yes I'm very happy with it. They're presented for different reasons, though. One is making statements about the Aboriginals and the whites, as we discussed. In *Barbarosa*, because it was a relationship picture, the camera was in on the faces all the time – the landscapes were their faces and I was in there and that's what I was examining. I kept reminding you that this very intimate thing was taking place in this unbelievably harsh environment.

You use an interesting device to represent the passing of time, with the passage of the sun reflected on the landscape.
Yes. If you look at that carefully it's not chronological. It's sort of mystical, to say that there's something else going on. We used the same technique near the start, when Barbarosa and Karl, his sidekick, meet and they ride across the landscape. The light where they're riding doesn't change, but behind them the colour and light changes about four or five times. Now I did that and I bet that nobody ever noticed it but I bet they got a kind of unsettling feeling. It was to create a mythical atmosphere.

Someone described the movie to me as an exploration of the nature of myth.
That's correct. The film that Bill Witliffe wanted to make was the hairy underbelly of a myth. One of the big lessons for me was that you don't necessarily have to specifically point to a myth, or something

you're trying to say. If you direct everything with that in mind, everybody's reactions to a person, the way that person does things and so on, it comes through. It is never overtly stated, but it still comes through.

In the end Karl, the sidekick, takes over the role of Barbarosa. Barbarosa has warned Karl against the lifestyle, yet seems to trap him into it. What is the film's attitude to the transformation?
Great. The myth's got to go on. Karl has lost everything. The only thing he's got now is that family and Barbarosa's daughter. He's understood his relationship with the family and the family's relationship with him and he likes it. He's a rogue. It's also saying something about the peculiar morality of that savage time and environment: he thinks that family is terrific. I don't, but he does.

I think one of the best sequences is where Barbarosa and Karl are climbing up what looks like a sheer cliff face. There's a moment of surprise when Karl accidently grabs a rattlesnake and falls back into the river below.
That was shot in the Big Ben National Park. They were over 400 metres high, those cliffs, and it was very hard to get that on film because I had nothing beneath to give any perspective. Actually we had another stunt planned there originally, which we couldn't do for budgetary reasons. When Bill came up with having Gary Busey accidentally grab the snake, we all said 'oh, not the bloody rattlesnake in the hole. What the hell, we'll just make it a little more exciting.' It is amazing rigging on the snake. That is special effects at its best. There were people operating its tail, and its head and its shooting forward. They deserve the credit for that one. The sound effects on that are quite remarkable too. We had a very brilliant guy here working on sound. When the snake is thrown away, he has taken a snake's hiss and played it in reverse at a slightly higher speed so that you feel it going away from you. He knew that he had to have a real snake's hiss because there is a certain quality in it no matter which way you play it. In fact the sound effects in the whole picture are quite remarkable. At the beginning of the film when Gary Busey is going through the thorns and he is getting ripped and scratched, there are whips, there are drums bumbling in there. There is amazing stuff that you don't

hear but you feel it. There are fourteen different kinds of wind in that film – in all the quiet passages where you think it's just silence, there's a wind that's doing something for you.

How did you find working with the American actors – you were talking earlier about actors becoming too self important. Is the star system something that you found difficult to adjust to in Hollywood?
It can be. They play power games and they want things done their way. Willie Nelson I found very eager to learn and develop his acting, and very good at receiving directions and giving things back. Gary Busey is a very instinctive actor who arrives at the point of performance by creating aggravation in everybody. That's his way of getting there and there is something of a star complex there, which I think is a shame because it prevents him from reaching even greater heights as an actor. The performance in some cases is in spite of his behaviour, but he always knew his lines and he knew what he was doing and why. He is a very good actor, he could just go about it in a way that's slightly easier on everybody. He was startled himself by how good some of what he did was, but I am the first director he hasn't destroyed. And that costs you in a film. It's a pity, because a picture is not just about an actor, or a cameraman, or a director, it's about everything combining. And to destroy that because you want the camera in on your eyes, or you don't want to come out, or you're throwing a tizzy for some reason or other – that is crazy, and I think it's sad. We had to change the way we work, and sometimes other things were lost.

You have said that Barbarosa *was the film where your craft was developed more than any other. What do you mean by that?*
Just a greater technical surety, better application of particular things in my approach. Under some of the pressures I had Ian Baker, my cameraman, hauling me back to some of those things, which was very helpful. He helped me formulate my approach. For example, we used long lenses a lot, even on dialogue sequences, which is what made the faces become the landscapes and pushed everything else into strange patinas. And I learnt some things about stories – about people needing goals, places to arrive at and go to, about forward motion in a picture, and about the emotional drive taking over at a specific point

and pushing through to a conclusion as quickly as possible without introducing diverting information. I learnt a lot of that from the difficulties in the picture.

REFLECTING ON DIRECTING
The Look of the Films

Do you think that Australian films have a recognisable look?
To a certain extent, but I think that's because of the light of the country. There are a lot of commercial cinematographers who understand about painting and still photography, the use of back light, or exposing light for the shade on the face so that the background burns out, because that is the look of the country. The light varies in different countries. For instance, we don't have the strange clear light that the Swedes have – that very whitish pure light. The local light dictates a lot of what you do or what you pick up on if you're good at it, whether it is the haze, the colours on a specific day, or the folds in the hills.

The Devil's Playground *certainly captures the winter light around Melbourne very clearly.*
The Devil's Playground was pretty unique at the time because we used very little lighting. We gave ourselves a lot of agony using very fast lenses, which give you very little depth of focus, but mean you can light a match and have the light just explode on the actor's face. The sequence in the hotel is the best example of that. We wanted the film to look not lit, to look as natural as if you just walked into the room. Somebody said as an insult after they saw *Libido*, 'they didn't even light the bloody thing.' I turned around and said 'thank you very much.'

Thoughtfully composed shots and images are a hallmark of your films. Do you feel that you learned lessons in advertising about ways of putting things on the screen that were carried over into film?
Sure. In commercials I had a chance to experiment with groupings, with positionings, which I see now in good theatre, ballet, and

paintings. Groupings are a terrific, dynamic thing, and I was able to play with elements like that. Also to shoot through things: I like a very wide frame because then I can shutter it down to the format that I want or explode it out by using objects that relate to what's going on, but block the camera's view. Ian Baker and I like doing that without using optical effects. The experience with positioning of things, the use of negative space, the working against white helped me a lot. That and working with good designers. I don't like doing production shots: every shot has got to be advancing the story in some way or making a point, so that I am not just saying 'here we are in this beautiful country.' I am saying 'how small these people are in this country' or 'how isolated that person is,' as well. I think that is important, and I like to set something up at one stage that will make a point later.

The Family

The idea of the family is very much the centre of Jimmie's experience and of his war with white society, and one of the primary things that drives him over the edge is the fact that his wife gives birth to a white child; it's not his child. I was wondering how important a theme the family is for you – I heard you had planned once to make a film about a man who jumps off the Gap, Sydney's famous suicide spot, taking his two children with him.

I remember reading that when I was about sixteen and being horrified, absolutely horrified. What did those children think on the way down? What possessed that man? I've read variations of that about six or seven times a year, and it's always written up that the guy was a wonderful guy and they used to walk around holding hands – bullshit. I started writing it but I had to stop, it disturbed me too much. I wanted to take four people who knew one another, who all went off successfully or unsuccessfully into different walks of life. They all had quite similar personalities because of their attraction to one another, and I wanted the film to change from house to house, mid-conversation, so you wouldn't be sure which house you were in. I wanted to say that in every one of us, there's a baby basher, or a murderer. I wanted to examine it because I wondered how could you ever, ever do that, and because maybe the man at the Gap wondered that himself one day, and somehow everything crushed in on him. Why did he take them with him? Guilt at leaving them behind? Disgust at the world and not wanting them to have to go through it? Revenge? I think there are about eight reasons why he would do it, but I dropped the subject. You really had to go too far into regions that I didn't want to get into.

There's a family in The Devil's Playground *too. The scene where Tom goes off to a picnic with his family is a quite idealised picture of family life.*
He was away from the institution, in the bosom of his family. It was just an unthreatening, comforting, secure, pleasant family visit. It's just meant to be warm. It gains in contrast to everything else, too.

Families can be seen as constricting as well.
They can be, and I'm sure they are by a lot of people at certain ages. But it's also who you are closest to and most relaxed with, in a way. If you're looking for whether I've got a thing about families, no.

The   Press

Were you bitter about the reaction to Jimmie Blacksmith *in Australia.*
I was disappointed, naturally. I expected some of it, as I explained. I was very angry at some members of the film industry who chose to use public criticism of the film to further their own careers in some way or another. I think that's despicable and it shows a lack of intelligence because one of the most successful things about Australian cinema is the way the better people in it help one another and understand that if any one of us is successful and breaks down barriers, it makes it easier for the rest of us. As regards the press reaction, no. They are opinions and everybody's entitled to their opinions and while you might be disappointed and have hoped for a better reaction, it's nothing to be bitter about.

How important to you is public recognition?
I know what I've done, what I haven't done, what I would like to do and how far I have to go, so it doesn't matter. I mean it's nice but I separate those things, and I don't get excited or angry when I read anything in the press because to me that's commodity time. I'm a commodity and that press space helps sell the picture. I divorce myself from it because I think you can fool yourself into thinking you're somebody that you aren't. I just happen to be a person who directs films. I direct films because I have a lot of feelings about life that I would like to express. I also see film as fun and entertainment – I'd like to do musicals, sheer fun things as well. It just happens that for some reason this is what I can do and I enjoy it and I am learning all the time. So that doesn't make me anybody special, it just makes me a bloke who makes films.

The   Role   of   the   Director

Do you see yourself as an artist?
Probably I'd like to. Yes, I do, but not in a pompous way. I certainly don't see myself as just churning out stuff. I would like to make as many films as I can that deliver a new experience, though that's not always possible.

How do you see the role of the director working in the team?
A good director is open to surprises and enhancement from the actors and the crew, providing that happens along the lines of the discipline and design of the film. Those people are not just there to supply you with what you've already imagined. Hopefully the crew members are as talented in their area as you are in yours, and they will take you somewhere further. That's where the real role of the director comes in, because he is the focus of all the talents, the one who directs everything between the riverbanks. The director is the one who is responsible for the vision in that he makes sure everybody contributes to a specific end. But of course directors work in extraordinarily different ways. A lot of directors don't direct camera at all, and know nothing about the camera, or lighting or lenses. Then a lot of directors do camera only and never tell the actors what to do.

That's the biggest complaint I've heard in the US, that actors don't know what they're doing because they're not being directed or told. Then there is the system in America where the stars won't do what the directors tell them, and that's untenable as far as I'm concerned.

It's often remarked that there's at least the appearance of a lot more democracy on Australian film sets than American ones.
Nonsense, total nonsense. What that might come from is that Australians don't think they have bosses. Now that's okay, but some people do necessarily have positions of authority and maybe the lines of demarcation are more clearly drawn in Hollywood. In America people call you 'sir', but they call any head of department 'sir', and they call their fathers 'sir' – so I don't think it's 'sir' in the way it's used in England. Nobody does that in Australia and everybody eats together and does things together and is a closer kind of group. But that's phony in one respect – underneath it all it really isn't any different. Directors might seem to be nice blokes in Australia, but they're not really. I know most of them and they want what they want.

Which directors do you particularly admire?
A long list. Kurosawa and a lot of the other Japanese directors: Mizoguchi, Ozu, Oshima. I like the English directors from the kitchen-sink, new wave era – *Look Back in Anger* and so on. As much as the directors, there was a school of writing that came out at that time. I tend to name directors, because that's what I knew about at the time, but a lot of the credit should go to the writers. I think writers are very badly forgotten – the basis of all films is the script; if the script isn't good you don't have a good film. I like the Czechs – Jiri Menzel is still there, making the most charming, whimsical films, and Milos Forman and Ivan Passer are in the US. I like Satyajit Ray from India, Luis Bunuel from Spain, now Mexico, and I liked the French and the Italians who came out at the same time. Of the American directors there's John Huston; I like a lot of his films: *Fat City, Treasure of The Sierra Madre.* I'm not a John Ford fan, though. I like Bob Fosse; I think Woody Allen is sensational; Billy Wilder I love; and William Wyler. Often it is the actors you remember from those films, like Hepburn and Tracy, and Clark Gable and Claudette Colbert.

AN AUSTRALIAN OR MID-PACIFIC CINEMA?

Working in Hollywood

Having been a fan of European films as much as of American films, what did coming to Hollywood mean for you?
Nearly everybody comes to Hollywood at some time or another, because in the end it is through here that you are chanelled out to larger markets. Hollywood as it was doesn't exist; now it is an international centre for filmmaking: the Germans, the Brazilians, and the English are here. Some of them can come to terms with it and stay and some of them can't and want to go back to their own culture. There are two reasons for that: one is because they can only express themselves in their own culture, which is fair enough; the other is because they are unable to contend with the system here. The system can crucify people on the one hand and yet on the other hand it can squeeze them until they are so refined they come up with something that is beyond what the system expects, without them losing any integrity. I came here for that pressure cooker.

What are you actually talking about when you talk about that brutality?
It is very like the things I used to complain about in advertising, where there were account executives who weren't necessarily skilled in advertising, who were representing a brand manager who wasn't necessarily skilled, who was representing a marketing manager, who was representing the company. And none of these people really had the power to say anything; they had all become corporate people who were subservient to someone who was subservient to someone else, so they weren't game to take chances or make decisions. They were only empowered to say 'no', and they only did that with a certain amount of trepidation. They feel they've got to contribute, so instead of being able to recognise that a person is going to give you something unusual, and saying 'this creative guy has made three extraordinary successes out of ten, let him do whatever it is he does', they have got to squeeze it into some package where they can understand it, have some control on it and contribute to it. And in the

process they are brutalising it and crushing out all the creativity.

They won't do something that is completely different, because how do they know it is going to work? So they do the films from the past. Nobody thought *E.T.* was going to be a success. Nobody thought *Star Wars* was going to be a success and I have got to tell you, they gave those people hell. There are no showmen in Hollywood now. I would rather go up against Jack Warner who I hear was an absolute brute, or Harry Cohn, or any of those people, because they were showmen. They were out there and they were saying, we are doing this for this reason and that reason. You can face that, you can go in and attack that; you can't attack nebulous negativism.

Have you had much personal experience of this sort of thing?
Yes, I have, in the number of projects that I believe are very worthy that have fallen through. I've got an adult comedy, quite sophisticated and yet very funny, with three current stars prepared to be in it. But I cannot get it made because the current philosophy refers to the 'comic-strip pictures', and unless it is 'high concept' or an 'event' picture, or they're using a new word now, 'soft' – they won't make it. And that's happened to me with five or six different projects.

Just explain those terms. What is 'high concept'?
I don't know, I have no idea. If you work them out, let me know. They're just the fashionable words at the moment. I have had films at studios and the studio executives change. A new studio executive is not going to pick up the work of the guy who's just been fired, so he kills the project. So you take it somewhere else and they want changes to the script, until eventually what you've got is another script altogether, and suddenly you think 'just a minute, I'm not doing the film I set out to do, I'm just doing a film that these people want, what am I doing this for?' So you say 'sorry, this is over, finished, I'm going,' and then they get upset, and you say 'well, too bad, I want to make my film, not the one you have reduced it to.' That has happened to me a number of times.

When I took on *Barbarosa*, I hunted around and I found a location I thought was perfect. It had roads everywhere and you could work in a 360° circle at any time of the day. You could make a scene work with that great light, give it texture and quality – none of which they understood. And they tried to jockey me out of it. They said it was impossible because it was too expensive, so I dropped it and looked at some other areas. They weren't good enough so I made some more enquiries and found out it wasn't impossible at all – the production manager was telling me that it was impossible simply because there was not enough accommodation. I said 'I can't make the picture, I'm finished.' I eventually did it because they said 'you can't leave,' and I said 'well, I can't make the picture unless you get rid of the production manager and you give me my location.'

Decisions are made on the basis of money but they are often incorrect. You might save twenty cents an hour on some person but he might cost you $250, so you have to say 'I don't want that person, I want this person who is more expensive because it is ultimately going to be cheaper.' In the end you have no recourse but to resign, otherwise you end up with a stinking picture. And no one is ever going to remember what they did to you, they are only going to remember what they see on the screen, and your name is on it.

The executives are mostly business people who have no practical experience in the film business. They did not grow up through the industry, knowing the departments and who does what and why and how you save money, so they make the wrong decisions. Everything is about the deal, and who can be packaged for what, and what actors can get you this or that.

Almost the least important part of the process it seems, is making the film. That is, until you get all the people together and you are working – because if you have managed to batter through good people, they are sensational. They give as much as you give, they are as creative in what they do as you are and they make things so easy that it's a joy. You walk on to a set and there is a fire there and you think 'where did that come from, I didn't see that.' Somebody has dug holes, planted gas things, done all that without you even seeing it, and it is where you had always wanted it to be. They are inventive, they are giving you extra stuff all the time. Dolly pushers will give me parameters: 'If you want this or this, I need more notice. If you want anything else, just tell us and we will do it like that.' So you are free not to worry about whether you can do a dolly or not. Then when you do a tracking shot that might be three minutes long, the guy pushing the dolly is listening to every word of the dialogue and he is varying his speed so that he reaches the spot he has to reach right on the word he has to reach it every time. I found that joyous, I found that just extraordinary: they care and they keep caring and there is no real bitching. There is some crude stuff to do with when we have lunch and so on, but basically they are there to work and that's what they do.

Hollywood and Australia

Is it different from Australia?
Different only in that they have had a lot more experience, so the knowledge is increased, but I am sure that is growing in Australia. In general the crews in Australia were a little inexperienced, a little clock conscious, a little TV production conscious, a little non-understanding of anybody who tried to work differently, and the morning and afternoon tea breaks and things like that are a killer. But I worked with a good Hollywood crew, and I think here, just like in Australia now, there aren't that many good crews. But I do miss things about working in Australia – it's simpler. In Australia, you get the script, and that's what you want to make, and all your energies and all your excitement go towards getting that made. Here, there's such frustration, you're almost venomous by the time you're making the picture – you have to get over that hatred of the process you've been through to get back into the joy of making the film. It's a purer intention in Australia, and I think it shows.

What sort of concessions do you have to make to a Hollywood lifestyle?
Well, I've been living here for three years, and I don't make any. I do not like the lack of focus in Los Angeles, of having no city centre. It takes a while to adjust. There are some great things here but it is an industry town.

Do you have to go to film-business cocktail parties?
I don't do any of that. Occasionally I might, but I don't like most of those people, I don't like talking business all the time. That is what is

wrong with the joint. I would much rather live in a society where my
friends are outside the business as much as inside, or more, so that
you are in contact with life and real people. Apart from having a richer
life, a less insulated existence, that is where your material comes
from.

You said in Playboy *that Americans are as different from
Australians as the French are, but that it took you a while to
recognise that. What did you mean?*
Humour, attitudes, expressions. You're fooled that the English
language is a common bond, but it isn't. The very way you say
sentences – some of the strangest words you think are common are
not common. The humour, the irreverence, the offhandedness and
the laconic thing that Australians have is totally misunderstood here.
You think you are being funny and people are getting insulted and
vice versa. They praise you – 'you have such wonderful talent' and all
that. In Australia it just makes you cringe, you sit there thinking,
please go away. On one level they are able to express themselves with
far more lucidity than we do, but on the other level you have to think,
do they really mean that?

Do you feel integrated into LA now?
No, I miss the footy.

Do you see yourself going back to Australia?
I'd like to live between both countries. My intention was to come to
America and do a few films in a row, applying what I've learnt, getting
a different perspective and hopefully getting a name for myself, which
would then help me market my Australian films. I have some subjects
that I really want to do in Australia, but I wanted to get some more
experience, to get a little more facility before I tackled them.

Has it been worth it financially to come to America?
Not in the least. Not yet. It may be, but it's very expensive to live here
and that's compounded by the fact that I have to go to Australia a lot.
It sounds like you are receiving a lot of money, but that money is like
turnover to a business, because you have agents and lawyers and
accountants, and Directors' Guild and Writers' Guild fees and all of

those things. If you crack it lucky, terrific. If a film makes a lot of money then you might see something, and of course as you make more films your price goes up – but by that time I might want to go home and do a film. It has been expensive. I have held out for almost two years. I have refused a lot of films and for a lot of money. Thems the breaks – I probably wouldn't have done them well, anyway. And in Australia I have my own production company, in partnership with other people. I have a base and an organisation and I do everything through that and it works. Here I am an individual and I go from place to place, and continually have to re-establish who does what. As well, I am a little torn about writing. I hope my next film will be written by me. You work differently when you work on your own things, though it's very valuable to work on other peoples' projects as well, just to make sure that you are applying the same objectivity to your own. You definitely come to understand your own work better.

Has the quality of your passion for filmmaking changed while you've been in Hollywood?
Nope. The frustrations have become a little greater, but mostly it's just different. You have to have an extraordinary amount of energy just to get through to make a film – it's a year out of your life, so you better like the damn thing. I have to be really attracted to the film. I've turned down a lot because I just don't feel for them, and I don't want to do remakes. I have so many films I'd like to do and so many things I want to say, it's a waste. But it's my hobby too – I enjoy it.

An Australian Identity

What is there about Australia that you are interested in expressing?
Lots of things. Mostly it has to do with expressing things with our voice, our humour, our irreverence, our naiveté if you like. I would be interested in doing a film about Norman Lindsay, because he is a study of whether an artist should go overseas or stay at home. Also the question of 'is near enough good enough?' interests me. How much effort should you put into something: should you put 100 per cent effort in to come up with an 80 per cent result, or should you put

in an 80 per cent effort to come up with a 70 per cent result and get on
with life. They are very valid questions in Australia, an extension of
'she'll be sweet' or 'she'll be right' if you like. What is right? What
kind of world do we want? Somebody said to me 'Australia nearly had
a revolution when Whitlam was thrown out of power'. I said 'what
for?' While we might have apathy and a certain amount of
unemployment and poverty, in general we are so much better off than
almost any other country. What is it that we want out of life, given
where we came from? Do we want anything more than to lie in the sun
and eat prawns and have a good time? I think that has to be
examined.

What do you think?
I think it's a combination. I think we are probably too sophisticated
now. I think we definitely have to have pursuits of the mind, and a bit
of drive and enthusiasm, energy and eccentricity, but not to the
elimination of enjoying nature and the good things, like sitting in the
sun and enjoying companionship and those much maligned
Australian pursuits.

Is there an identifiable Australian character that interests you?
Specifically, no. In general, yes. I would like to do something about
migrants in Australia, and about Australia's position in Asia and the
influence of Asia. I'd like to do the story of Peter Allen, the
entertainer, as a story of working in the clubs, a bittersweet musical
which could be quite different.

*How do you feel about the presentation of sexuality in Australian
films? Would you agree that in general it's something we don't do
very well?*
Gee, I hope I do it well. I think the sex in *Jimmie Blacksmith* is
terrific. I think perhaps some of our early films were a little too
exploitive and straining to be erotic. I think being erotic is actually a
lot easier than that, because it's a textural thing you can do in a film.
And I don't think many of our subjects have really given us that
opportunity – I think, fortunately, that most of us have avoided being
exploitive and dropping it in just for the sake of titillation or
commerciality. If it is part of the story and is essential to the story, it

goes in, and if it isn't, it doesn't. In George Miller's film *Mad Max 2 (The Road Warrior),* the dog and the woman get killed. That doesn't happen in Hollywood because they are looking at it from a purely commercial standpoint. We don't care; we follow the dictates of the story, and I think that's a great plus. But it's true that we haven't really explored sexuality; maybe we are still a little embarrassed. When an Australian says 'I luv ya', it's not quite as romantic as 'je t'adore'. It reflects the way Australians deal with sex – there's a tendency to be a little blunt, I think.

What are the qualities about Australian cinema that you like?
It isn't always there, but it's the freshness of approach, the openness, and the unabashed honesty. It's Australian in what you are looking at, in the way it's photographed, in the way it's written, and the way it is structured, in the acting and the humour. The better films are the films that have an indigenous subject matter, that are by us and about us, and with us. They may have a universal theme but they are our point of view and they're different. The films I don't like and the films I believe have failed are the ones that have sopped to the international market, either with international stars or international themes or subjects – pseudo-American horror pictures or pseudo-American thrillers or whatever. It's nonsense; you are not going to do that better than the Yanks. I think that our films are refreshing; they are simple without being simplistic. But I certainly don't think they are all so very wonderful. I think too few people working in film care enough about using the medium to its fullest – sound, picture, composition, cutting – all of which can be used differently, can avoid being formularised.

Can you think of examples of where that Australianness is evident?
It permeates the whole picture: you can't pick out specific examples because it relates to structure, it relates to delivery of lines, it relates to body movement, it relates to the whole pacing of the picture, the lack of formula. You can't zero in on a point and drag it out, it's not there to do. There are obvious things – our light is very different, the bush is very different, but not all our pictures are about the outdoors. Our houses, our homesteads, our clothing in the period things are all

very different. Pioneering against harsh environments, survival, all of those things. But that is very obvious and that's not what it is. It is in the way people think and speak and react. It is the whole tone of it. *Breaker Morant* is possibly the easiest and best example of all of that, and so is *Gallipoli*. It is in the very fibre of the picture – you're laughing and there is no joke on the screen, you are just laughing because it's so true to the way people behave, and that's terrific. That comes from the writing.

The Director as Addict

Are you a person who gives 80 per cent for a 70 per cent result?
No, I give everything. I try not to let it take up my personal life, though, I think that's silly. But when I'm going, I'm going.

How do you find that balance?
Trial and error. I don't know the answer to that. I may not have found it. Just make sure you keep them with you, make sure there are times when you are not working and you stop and take stock and give time. It's all-consuming, it demands a lot of time. When you are shooting, you get four hours sleep a night and probably no days off. And the period leading up to that is pretty tough as well.

The critic Pauline Kael talks about a quality of obsession that she says great filmmakers have and she includes you among those. Do you feel obsessed?
You've got to be, I guess. I was going to say before when we were talking about Australia and whether you should have beer and prawns and sit in the sun – maybe some of us are cursed with culture. Maybe we should just relax and sit in the sun and have decent conversations. That's where it all came from originally. But yes, it is an obsession. I have a million things that I want to do and a lot of things that I want to learn, and a lot of films I want to make, and I am just starting.

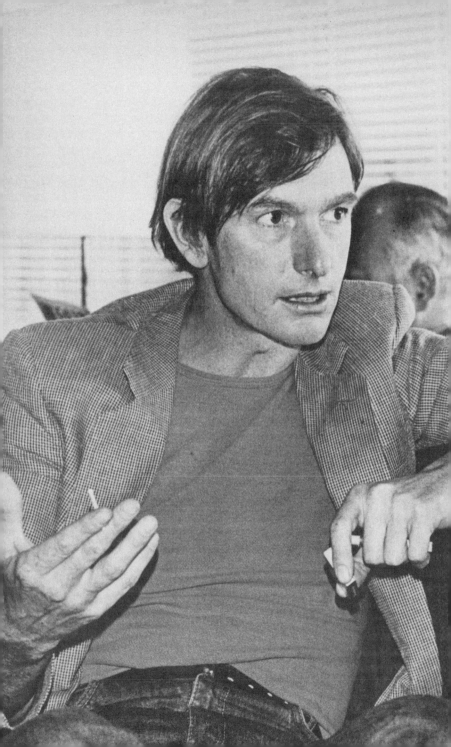

PETER WEIR

'*Gallipoli* was my graduation film,' says Peter Weir. It was then, he believes, that his technique caught up with his inspiration. Inspiration is central to Peter Weir's filmmaking: his approach is intuitive rather than cerebral. It is almost a point of honour with him.

Weir's first two films, *Homesdale* (1971) and *The Cars that Ate Paris* (1974), were quirky black comedies, developments of the amateur revues he had been staging in his spare time. *Picnic at Hanging Rock* (1975) and *The Last Wave* (1977) were more conscious attempts to deal with the fragility of commonsense reality, with the recognition that 'within the ordinary lies the extraordinary'. *Picnic at Hanging Rock,* based on the Joan Lindsay novel about the unexplained disappearance of a group of schoolgirls in the last century, was a turning point in the development of the new cinema in Australia: it was the first Australian film that was clearly a 'quality film'. Weir became the first Australian 'auteur' as *Picnic* legitimated Australian movies for the middle-class audience still ready to believe in the inferiority of Australian culture.

Picnic and especially *The Last Wave*, about a lawyer who finds himself psychically drawn to a group of Aboriginals he is defending, reflect Weir's interest in theories of myths and dreams. A concern with ideas and experiences that were outside the realm of common-sense everyday understanding was shared by many people in the sixties. Like many young people at the time Weir was very influenced by the new ways of thinking, and was a strong opponent of the war in Vietnam. Weir's award-winning *Michael*, one section of the 1970 film about youth called *Three To Go*, produced by the Common-wealth Film Unit, is a classic statement of some of those values.

A lapsed radical – 'I detest dogma' – Weir nonetheless remains faithful to some of the attitudes of the era. 'Just because the decade ends doesn't mean we stop wondering about the enormous gap between the Third World and our world; we don't stop thinking about love or about how to construct some sort of moral system,' he says. He is profoundly individualistic: 'I always marched in the nonaligned section of the anti-war marches,' he affirms, and he is emphatic that his interest in mysticism does not extend to cults that demand abandoning independent thought and action.

Though they came to the conclusion by different routes, Weir shares with George Miller the opinion that 'greater detachment is ultimately a freedom' for a director. Aside from making you more vulnerable to the sting of critical rejection, working to intuition rather than to plan can threaten the coherence of a film, as the director risks losing control. After some experimentation Weir has moved away from the 'exhilaration' of extreme openness and spontaneity on the set. There is the danger too of 'the filmmaker as god', in Weir's phrase: in placing him or herself at the centre of the work the director can grow self-obsessed, and the audience's view can also become unbalanced, the director being seen as some kind of guru.

In *Gallipoli* (1981) Weir employed a more structured approach than before, but his distinctive sensibility did not disappear. The luminous shots of the pyramids under which the Australian soldiers camp on their way to the Turkish battlefield are arguably more potent evocations of the dislocation of past and present, the eternal and the everyday, than the more pointed mysteries of *Picnic at Hanging Rock* and *The Last Wave*. In *The Year of Living Dangerously* (1982), adapted from Christopher Koch's novel about the coup of the Indonesian generals that toppled Sukarno in 1965, there is a harmonious integration of the imagery of the traditional wayang puppets into the substance of the story. *The Year of Living Dangerously* sets a fine romance in an authentically turbulent Indonesian setting, the great events of the time moving just beyond the grasp of the Westerners who are the film's subjects. As in *Gallipoli* Weir's interest is in the people rather than the events; his concern is with personal rather than political morality. For some it is his most successful film yet; others are frustrated by the diversity of its concerns and the absence of a clear political stance.

Financed by the giant American MGM movie corporation but produced in Australia by long-time Weir associates Hal and Jim McElroy, *Living Dangerously* represents one way for a director to work with the American film industry without having to move to foreign territory. The 1980 *Gallipoli* also represented a new approach to financing, being funded entirely by expatriate moguls Rupert Murdoch and Robert Stigwood through their Associated R & R Films.

Weir's personality is clearly stamped on his films, yet he appears to be less engaged in the construction of individual shots than some directors; he prefers to collaborate with a trusted camera operator and director of photography. An important contribution to the look of Weir's films has also come from Wendy Weir, the director's wife, who was credited as production designer on the 1979 telemovie *The Plumber*, and as design consultant on *Gallipoli* and *The Year of Living Dangerously.*

In conversation Weir has a youthful intensity, choosing allusive, literary phrases to capture nuances of feeling as he recalls the past. He is more comfortable talking publicly about events and stages in his life than in reflecting on more general issues and approaches, either to his own work or to the Australian cinema in general. This interview reflects that: in checking the transcript Weir excised many of the analytical and interpretive comments. His lucid, evocative grasp of language make him 'excellent copy', but Weir clearly finds public discussion of his work an ordeal. Though relaxed, direct and professional in the recording of this interview, agreement on the final transcript was difficult to reach and the published version is the last of several proposed revisions

Weir lives just north of Sydney in an old house overlooking a remarkable tree-framed view of sand and water. 'I don't really feel as if we own this,' he says, and you know what he means: it is a view almost too beautiful to be private property. The house has a comfortable yet slightly exotic air. Furnished with timber, bamboo and Asian fabrics its large windows make the interior seem continuous with the surrounding garden. Weir's study, apart from the house and past a small rock garden and waterfall he built himself, has a similar atmosphere. Volumes of war history and a collection of World War One helmets and weaponry are ranged a little incongruously alongside the novels on which his films have been based, and diverse works of fact, place and theory from Montezuma to the Australian Stony Desert.

Weir is one of the most successful of Australia's directors, both at home and overseas. He is polite and quietly spoken with a boyish look. A man of strong attractions and dislikes, he vehemently defends his films against criticism from those writers he labels 'academic' who expect a different sort of clarity from him, demanding that conclusions be drawn and answers be given. Such critics have, he says, a view of art and life so remote from his own that he doubts he will ever satisfy them: 'I can only wave across a distance,' he says, 'as the person heads in another direction.'

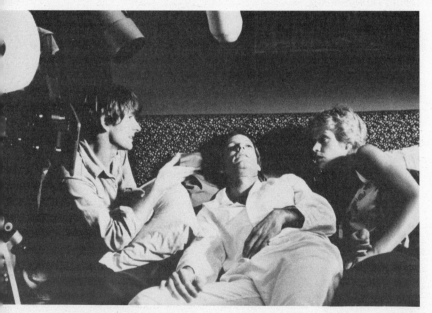

Above: Peter Weir directs Richard Chamberlain and Olivia Hamnett in *The Last Wave.*

Above right: 'I think I became fond of the people I satirized.'
From left to right, Anzacs Robert Grubb, Mel Gibson, David Argue and Tim McKenzie on the loose in Cairo in *Gallipoli.*

Below right: Bill Hunter (Major Barton) leads camera operator John Seale and crew through the trenches in *Gallipoli.*

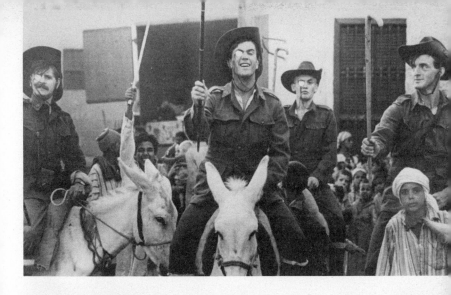

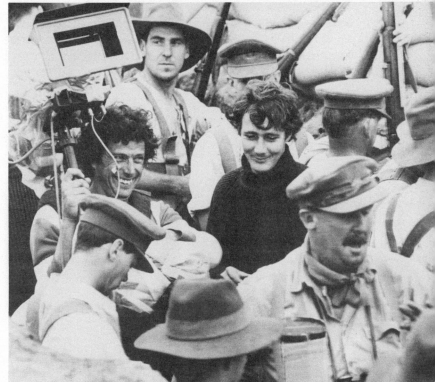

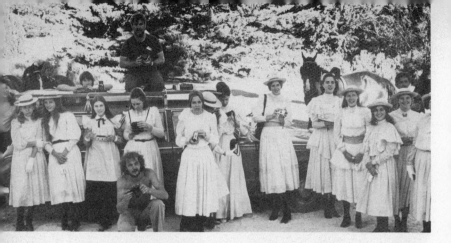

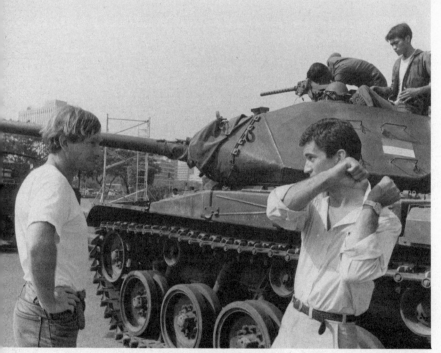

Above: 'We saw a couple of hundred girls in various states, but we found this particular pre-Raphaelite, nineteenth century look only in South Australia.' Farewell snapshot time on *Picnic at Hanging Rock.*

Below: Peter Weir, Mel Gibson (Guy Hamilton) and Indonesian army in *The Year of Living Dangerously.*

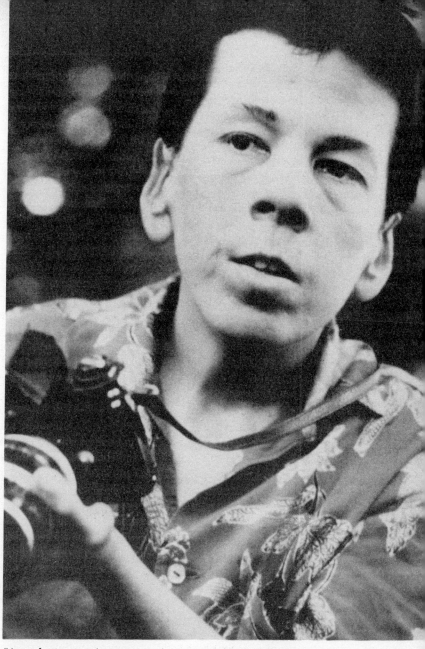

'Her performance is what matters.' Linda Hunt as Billy Kwan in *The Year of Living Dangerously*.

BEGINNINGS

Childhood

Sue Mathews: Where did you grow up?
Peter Weir: Sydney. We moved quite a bit until I was about twelve; my father was a real-estate agent and he would buy a house and move us into it for three or four years and then move us to another one. At one time we settled in Watson's Bay which was the beginning of a wonderful period. The settings are very exotic around there and I was fortunate enough to be brought up in the pre-television generation, so after school I'd be out in the streets. They'd be full of kids right through to dark; there would be balls bouncing and bits of things rolling down the street and neighbours chatting to each other and sitting outside, it was almost a village feeling. There was always a gang of kids: we would go over to the Glen and jump on trams as they went through, or explore caves that were supposedly Aboriginal, or go to the Gap which was nearby. There seemed to be a lot of danger, which I think adds so much to a child's life, the forbidden things that one shouldn't do or go near. When I was 12 we moved to Vaucluse. We were at the top of a little hill that led down to the park at Parsley Bay where there is a big suspension bridge. I was never out of the water, snorkling or spear fishing. Those years were linked with the water and the sea. I used to watch the ships going out, those huge liners going to Europe and from as early as I can remember I used to think that I'd like to be on one.

This was before television was introduced in Australia – did you have much contact with other areas of popular culture?
Comics! They were a big part of a kid's life, I used to collect them, swap them, sell them. I liked the Phantom and Scrooge McDuck – I always preferred him to Donald Duck – especially the ones that were about adventures in South America and Lost Cities. Then there were the pictures, the Saturday afternoon flicks. My father used to take me to the Wintergarden in Rose Bay. I loved Westerns, and the serials . . . it's interesting to see Spielberg and Lucas reproduce those for other generations.

Did your parents mind you collecting comics – did they feel you should be interested in other sorts of pursuits?
No, not really. From my earliest years I played very elaborate games. They took various forms, though they were generally war games, beginning with lead soldiers. There were very strict rules: if you got shot you really had to lie down, and you couldn't go 'pow', you had to make it sound like a gun. When I was twelve or thirteen, my parents became very concerned about these games, and had a talk with me, more or less saying that these sorts of games have gone on too long. I remember that conversation at the breakfast table really having some impact on me, and I moved onto other things after that.

Do you think that constructing those games was a precursor to an interest in making films?
Well, I think there is certainly a link between games and creativity. For example, many Japanese are very concerned because their children don't play anymore, it's all scholastic achievement from a very early age. My problem at school, however, was the study side. Actually I don't think I ever stopped playing games. In my teen years they took on a certain bizarre aspect. I would go to parties disguised as various characters – a visiting American student, a trainee priest, or a German merchant seaman. I very carefully rehearsed the friends who collaborated in these elaborate jokes. Most of them worked far too well and caused all sorts of problems, but they certainly livened things up.

Did you read novels?
I don't remember much reading. My father was a good storyteller, so when I was a young child, rather than reading a book before bed, my father would tell me stories. He had one enormously successful serial which ran for about two years. It was called *Black Bart Lamey's Treasure*, an exotic tale of the South Seas in the pirate days. I did read adventure stories – the Famous Five, Biggles, things that were popular in those times. Then when I hit secondary school, books were introduced as part of the examination process. I was one of those students who reacted extremely badly to that and saw reading books as a chore. It took me many years after I dropped out of university to get back to reading novels, and I've only just begun to get back to Shakespeare. Poetry I still can't touch.

Biggles and the Famous Five are English books – did you have a
sense of England as home or where we really belonged?
Not really. I do remember an intense period of interest in who we were
and getting out the family Bible and looking at some old photos. I was
astonished that our family hadn't kept any records of where we had
come from and who we were on either side of the family. I've asked
other Australians what records they have, and have found the same
story. A most extraordinary experiment in immigration: Anglo-
Saxon people who left the past behind, left their myths behind and
began again. It's helped me to understand why many of our films have
been period films, and why Australian audiences have been so drawn
to them – because of this need for myth.

How long ago did your family come to Australia?
I'm fourth generation – my great-grandfather and mother on both
sides were immigrants from England, Ireland and Scotland. I think
it's the Celt side that has come out most strongly.

Were you aware of things from America and things from England
as two separate sets of influences on Australia?
I was less aware of the English than of the Americans. In the fifties
American culture had a kind of exotic quality about it. I remember
once a friend of the family bringing us back long strips of chewing
gum, before we had that shape here. After 1956 I'd see odd American
television programmes and I was fascinated with those.

Were you aware of a tradition of Australian filmmaking?
Not really. I saw *Bush Christmas* and liked it, and I certainly loved
Charles Chauvel's *Jedda*, seeing it as a kid. I can still recall the
powerful highly coloured images from that film, but it was like
looking at a film from another culture. Everyone knew of the actor
Chips Rafferty. He *was* the industry in a way. A sort of one-man
band.

What about Australian literature?
I had very little interest in our literature and history – I always felt that
the grand events and the great adventures lay outside this country.

The image of that ship sailing out summed it up: the world lay elsewhere.

You've described your experience of literature at school as a fairly unhappy one – what was school like overall?
Well, the word 'unhappy' is something I've come to apply since. I was happy enough – but it was after school that things really began. I remember running down the hill, ripping my tie off and jumping on a tram and getting down to 'real life'. I went to a private school where the emphasis was on sport and academic achievement and I was not particularly good at either. I failed the Leaving Certificate and went to Vaucluse High where the atmosphere was very different. We had a history teacher called Bill Kneene who in the first class asked us to come up with our own ideas about the causes of the First World War. I recall that day very clearly: he was asking us to do our own research, telling us it mightn't be all known! Histroy came alive for me that day. Of course, we didn't find any illuminating facts, but from then on that year just took off and I passed and went on to Sydney University.

Rites   of   Passage: Uni   and   OS

It sounds like that was a more or less automatic transition?
It was what I wanted to do. I'd built up a picture of what university was going to be like. It was really a picture that might have been true in about the fifteenth century, you know, 'the student life', where we would all be singing and arguing into the night. But the first lecture I remember was on the novel *Portrait of the Artist as a Young Man*. I looked around and I couldn't believe it – there were 599 other people in this vast lecture theatre and an ant down the front with a microphone squeaking away for an hour about the meaning of the novel. I just looked at a couple of friends next to me and we all raised eyebrows and it wasn't too long before I was cutting those lectures and going to the pub.

I went to a poetry lecture where we'd been asked to read a Blake poem. I loved the poem and though we had to write something on it, I couldn't, I was so moved by the poem, so excited by it. I thought, well, it'll come out when we talk. Then in the classroom the lecturer put the poem on the board – it was very short – cut it up with his chalk into various sections and proceeded to introduce the seminar by saying 'this is really a poor example of Blake's work and a very bad poem for the following reasons . . .' I looked around and everyone was writing it down and I felt a flush come to the cheeks – I felt embarrassed that I had been moved by it. I didn't say a word during the whole thing and crept out – and began to cut those lectures too.

So I failed the first year, and pulled out and went into real estate. My father was glad I was out of University; he liked me getting down to business and earning some money. He had a one-man business and the plan was pretty clear that I would join him, and in the meantime get a couple of years' experience with other real-estate agents.

Working with other agents, not your father?
Yes, from about eighteen to twenty. I sold land. I went and visited all my blocks and made notes on them and then went back to the office. I remember the boss coming out and saying 'what are you doing?' I was ripping all those ones I didn't like out of the listing book. I said 'well, you can't sell something you don't think is any good.' Anyway I sold the lot and I'll never forget when I came in one morning and there was one of the other agents, ripping out all the houses in his book he didn't like. With the money I made I bought a one-way ticket to Europe with the intention of working in London, and set off on what was supposed to be a three or four months' visit.

How did it feel to be on a boat sailing out?
It felt like a beginning; I knew that whatever it was, it was going to happen.

You've said that the trip itself was quite a formative experience?
It was a Greek boat heading for Piraeus where it was due for a refit and as I came to know, when a ship is due for a refit, there is a kind of malaise amongst the crew. This affected the entertainment side of things and the Entertainments Officer had organised something like a fancy dress night, but not much else. So a few of us suggested a

ship's review and he said 'if you want to organise it, go ahead.' We also found a closed circuit TV on board – God knows what it was used for, but there was a little studio and TV sets in all the bars and some very bored passengers, so we asked if we could do a show.

On the TV?
Yes. We'd left Australia in the heyday of *The Mavis Bramston Show*, the Phillip Street Review, and Barry Humphries, so we did a kind of review format of satire and interviews with passengers. We got off the ship pale – we used to live in that little studio.

Did being in Europe alter your perspective on Australia significantly?
It was such an innocent time to travel – a time that was about to come to an end, as the ship voyages were about to end. It's one of those things that I responded to in Christopher Koch's book about 1965. You could draw a line through that year: it was a beginning and an end; it was the end of the 50's. It was just prior to the hippie wave and every young person hitching was a student.

One evening in Spain I was dropped off towards sunset and climbed a hill with some bread and wine. And during that evening it struck me very strongly that I was a European, that this was where we had come from and where I belonged. That was probably the beginning of an interest in thinking about immigration to our country and where we were in the world. Those of us who went to Europe for the first time by ship were very lucky – that understanding of the distance, of just how far away we were from our culture.

Were you working in England?
I was there for ten or eleven months. I had various jobs – grocery driver, lifeguard. They were great days – a feeling of optimism, of change, a wonderful period to be in London. In fact, it's always been difficult to go back. It was like a membership in a giant club, just to be young. 1965 – it was 'Flower Power', anti-Vietnam marches, rock and roll, and 'swinging London', as it came to be known. It was a feeling that I carried back with me and no doubt it contributed to my decision not to go back into real estate but to do any sort of work until I could get a job in television.

T e l e v i s i o n   a n d   V i e t n a m

Did you come back with a clear plan of working in films?
No. There was no film industry. And somehow with the optimism of
the sixties there was a feeling that everything was going to work out,
that you didn't need to plan. I knew I vaguely wanted to get into the
entertainment business – writing or acting, but I had no clear idea.
Television was the biggest employer, but it took several months
before I could get a job. Eventually I was taken on as a stagehand at
Channel Seven.

During this period I'd begun producing amateur revues. I'd
decided I wanted to do a revue at Christmas in 1966. So I got together
the nucleus of my old school friends. I found a little church hall we
could hire and we put on a revue called *A Little Night of Etc.* I
directed it and wrote a lot of the sketches.

What was Channel Seven like at the time?
Seven was the only station doing Australian drama at the time. They
had *My Name's McGooley* which was a very slick show for its time. I
liked working on that. Then they did *You Can't See Round Corners*
and *Motel* – they were really gambling on Australian drama, rather
than purchasing American shows. It was a wonderful period to be
there. In 1967 I decided to make a film for the Channel Seven Staff
Social Club Xmas Revue I'd been organising. It was called *Count
Vim,* and took a year to make and was about 15 minutes long. I think
they got a surprise at the station because they thought it was going to
be a comedy on funny characters around the place, the doorman and
the head of the Channel or something with funny hats on, but it
wasn't.

The station executives liked the film and asked if I wanted a job
directing the film sequence of what was then the last year of the
satirical revue, *The Mavis Bramston Show.* 1968 was a very tough
year because I really knew so little. I had to edit my own clips – it was a
very hard school to go through and a very good one. I used to cut the
original film which added to the tension – each time you made a splice
you had to be very careful not to damage the film or cut in the wrong
spot.

What sort of movies were you watching?
The commercial cinema. And I'd go to any of the 'underground' film screenings put on by Ubu films, the alternative film society at Sydney University – they took up *Count Vim* and put it in a program, *Underground '68* I think it was called. A film of Bruce Beresford's was shown too – he was working at the British Film Institute – and a couple of others who went on to do things, Albie Thoms being one. There was this magazine at the time called *Lumière*. It used to have a little section in every issue headed 'Australian Feature Film Production', with underneath it, 'Nil'. The next film I did for the staff club was *Buck Shotte*. I left someone else to do the revue in '68 and I made the film, which was much more elaborate in every way than *Count Vim*.

Did you do any writing for the Bramston show?
I was always submitting ideas and sketches. They took a couple, but mostly my stuff was considered too black. I continued to write, direct and perform in revue and film (working with Grahame Bond) until I saw the Monty Python show for the first time in 1971. At that point I decided to leave the revues and concentrate on film. When I saw that first show I thought 'they are better than we are' and I never wrote or acted in that sort of thing again.

Were you developing an interest in making films through going to the movies?
Not really. The films from overseas were big impressive productions – we didn't really make a connection between our 16mm films and the 35mm wide-screen film. A more important factor in the rebirth of the Australian film industry, I think, was the Vietnam War.

Was this through a rejection of American culture because of opposition to US foreign policy?
It wasn't as clear as against America, don't forget, because there was that tremendous kinship with, and borrowing from, the American anti-war movement. It was anti-establishment, and you saw one's own establishment as connected directly to the American establishment. It was very much about youth, really. A lot of it is embarrassing now in some ways – a lot of it is really very dangerous, I think. It

doesn't change one's view of what that war was and that what happened was right, but when you saw the Vietnamese cross over into Cambodia and earlier when you saw Pol Pot take over there, you found your so-called new-left views in tatters and realised how naive they were.

Had you become aware of Vietnam in England?
Oh yes, one of the friends I had met on the ship talked about Vietnam as much as he did about Dylan and marijuana; it was my introduction to these changes that were about to enter society.

How were the effects of the war and the film industry connected?
The war unleashed energy and conflict, passion. You always have to look at movements in society, to look at any sudden movement in the arts. You never get a sudden rash of painters, opera singers, dancers, or filmmakers just like that from nowhere. In this case it coincided with this great movement that I had become aware of overseas. Phrases were coined like 'do your own thing', 'the alternative society' – they've become clichés, but they had power then – and then there was the daily bombardment of songs, from Simon and Garfunkel to Bob Dylan and the Beatles. It was starting to come out of Hollywood with *The Graduate* and *M.A.S.H.*; even there a fresh direction was emerging.

It was a period of our own café society – there were groups of people meeting and talking and sharing ideas. And there were great changes happening in theatre – Bob Ellis and Michael Boddy wrote *The Legend of King O'Malley* which burst out on the scene as a fresh direction, and the underground films were happening through organisations like Ubu films. I think it came out of the passion in the streets, this feeling of a beginning and an ending, and somewhere people like Philip Adams and Barry Jones began to look around and see the potential, and to talk about government support for filmmakers.

Were you aware of this lobbying for a film industry?
No, and if I had been I probably wouldn't have been interested. It all sounded a bit too institutionalised for me, too formal or academic. Those ghosts of the university experience were still around. I liked

the life in the streets, I liked just music and laughter and talking, the camaraderie that was coming off that . . . I was suspicious of organisers like that at the time. It became a reality for me when my friends began to lose interest in giving up their Sundays. I was getting a little bit too organised, saying things like 'don't be late, learn your lines, the production manager will call you'. Production manager? I had begun to think about *Homesdale* and I was working on the script through '69 to '70. Somebody suggested that I apply to the Experimental Film Fund – Richard Brennan was the producer (he was at the Commonwealth Film Unit with me) and we worked out the budget to the last dollar. I think I was in the second batch of applicants and got $1912. It was a grant – I couldn't believe it: they *gave* it to you.

Why did you decide to leave Channel Seven?
Well, after a year of doing these film clips, in which they hadn't raised my salary, the Bramston show folded. I had a short holiday, and when I came back I found my name on the roster as a stagehand again. I went to the guy in charge and said 'you didn't give me a raise, and now you're just dropping me back' and he said 'that's right.' So I said 'I resign. Right now. I'm leaving today, goodbye.' He said 'fine, good luck.' I was out of work for months. I knew the only place I wanted to go then was the Commonwealth Film Unit. After about three months they took me on as a director.

The   Commonwealth   Film   Unit

Was there a sense of a community working towards a film industry at the Commonwealth Film Unit then?
It was like a film school and Gil Brealey and Richard Mason were our tutors. Gil had been in America and knew the way a film was made, knew about the simple formalities of constructing a script, of moving actors around, and so on. He ran a course for us really, and financed this with a series of Public Service Board training films. Some of the others there were Don Crombie, Brian Hannant, Arch Nicholson, who all became directors, and later Don McAlpine and Dean Semmler who went on to become leading directors of photography. I liked the atmosphere; it was the university that I had looked for in 1963. Gil

Brealey came up with the idea of *Three To Go* – three directors, three views of youth. My section was titled *Michael.*

Michael opens with a newsreel-style scene of tanks and soldiers in the streets of Sydney, then switches to the conservative young man Michael, in his everyday office job, and follows his attraction to a group of young people who represent freedom, anti-authority, humour – all those things that got called 'liberation'. How did you see the connection between that aspect of the counter-culture and the armed struggle you show at the start?
Those ideas of armed struggle were aspects of my own political naiveté and the naiveté of the times, but the anti-Vietnam war feelings had reached such a pitch in the late sixties that such speculation didn't seem out of the question.

It is interesting to see it now because it says so much about the times. The critique of conformity, for instance – you have some really funny things, like the line of businessmen waiting for the bus, all wearing the same suits and reading the same newspapers.
It was so simplistic, looking back. It's propaganda of the then 'new left', but of course why I'm embarrassed about a shot like that is you could have put someone as unconventional as Magritte in that line. We put so much emphasis on the outward display. In those days you could see someone with a beard and you could probably walk right up and start talking about how we should get out of Vietnam.

Later I remember getting caught out on that. I picked up a couple of hitchhikers who looked just as I did, jeans and long hair and so on. It must have been just before the end of the war and the Americans were launching their last offensive. There had just been news of a terrible bombing raid, and I said 'did you read that today – terrible, wasn't it?' And one of them said 'oh, the only solution is to nuke 'em.' It wasn't long after that John Lennon sang 'Let's get the hair off and see who's who.'

Another interesting thing in that film is the way you use rock music to tell the story.
In those days it was a substitute for dialogue. We didn't know how to

write dialogue for Australians and the actors were frightened of saying it. The sound of the Australian accent in films was totally unfamiliar. So I pulled a lot of tricks to have minimal dialogue in the picture. David Williamson had only just begun working in film at that stage. His influence spread later, as did that of other writers, like John Dingwall and Margaret Kelly – those who enabled us, or helped us, to speak.

In terms of technique, it's very much a montage approach with lots of fast editing and juxtaposing of images.
More so than was planned in the script. It was a case of the editor, Wayne Le Clos, helping me get out of a lot of trouble. Even though I had reached a reasonable technical level and the film won the prizes of the day, I didn't really know what I was doing. I was always one step ahead of myself, just charging right on out there and letting the techniques come after me. I still think that's the best way to go, and it certainly applied to all the early films, going right through until *Gallipoli* – that was my graduation film. The terrifying thing in those early films was not knowing why something *had* worked, even more than understanding why something *hadn't* worked.

I remember giving a lecture once to a media course. In the class before my lecture they were practising the various technical functions of a film crew. I watched them for a while and said 'what are they doing?' There was one group queued up in front of the camera, rather like divers on a diving board. One at a time they'd come forward and primp or make some movement at a certain spot and then go back to the end of the queue. 'They're practising hitting marks,' I was told. Other groups were writing up clapper boards, or dressing sets or something. 'I think it's important that they realise what an actor has to go through, in hitting marks, and performing,' the guy running the course said. I said 'if they've only got a two-year course, why waste time on something like that?' So I said to the students 'right, – let's get all this gear out of the way. This has got nothing to do with it, nothing. Let's just talk, about anything, everything, about stories, experiences. You've got too much of this gear. It's summoning up the ideas that's the hard thing – the inspiration, the passion. Without them, this stuff's useless.'

MAKING THE MOVIES

Homesdale

Homesdale *was a haunted house story, about a mysterious hotel or mental home. Where did the idea come from?*
It came from an old house we rented in several acres of land at Church Point. It was one of those properties that really had a story clinging to it. People would say as they came 'it reminds me of a hospital in the Crimea, with its wide verandahs and cream stucco.' I used to imagine rows of patients stretched out there recovering from their wounds. Others would say 'it's like a plantation house in South America.' It had a romance about it. 'A guest house' someone said and I remember we talked about guest houses and how, of course, they were going out of fashion by then, being replaced by motels. When I was young, some friends and I had gone up for a weekend and stayed at a place called Homesdale at Katoomba in the Blue Mountains. It had a dance and a host and hostess and was a very old-fashioned place. We'd gone up there under fictitious names pretending to be bank clerks on holiday or something. We got up to a lot of mischief. So *Homesdale* grew out of all that.

Homesdale *was your first film made outside the Commonwealth Film Unit. Was it a very chaotic experience?*
It was difficult. Also, I think it surprised friends in the cast and crew, because with the excitement of making this more complex film, we had come together with a very positive feeling. It was shot over a week and we were all living in the house or in tents in the grounds which didn't help because everyone had different hours – some liked to stay up till two drinking and playing guitars and others wanted to go to bed early. It was a highly organised film, which also contributed to the tension. But more importantly than that the subject matter of that film came onto the set as it has in all my films. It was a lot about mockery and bullying and nasty games of one kind or another and we lived and worked in that atmosphere.

Interlude

There was a four year interval between Homesdale *and* The Cars That Ate Paris, *what were you doing in that time?*
After *Homesdale* I went back to Europe on a grant from the Interim Council for the Film School. They were sending a lot of people around the world to study. England provided a breathing space and I spent my days on feature film sets out at Pinewood and Elstree, mainly working with special effects people. At the same time writing madly.

Scripts?
Yes. It was a great creative burst. We travelled through France and one day we came to a road block where there were some men standing in orange jackets with a portable 'Stop' sign. They said 'you can't go down here, you have to go back and use the side road.' I asked if it would link up to where I was going and they just said 'go'. It seemed rather odd, because there was no sign of any roadworks, just that little barrier. The detour led all over the place and it took us ages to find our way back. Why had I accepted the authority of the roadworkers? Probably because of their day-glo jackets, like the guy in a white coat is the doctor.

Weeks later in England, I saw a front page story in the paper about a shooting, some crime of passion, while down in a very small column was the fact that in Britain that weekend 23 people had lost their lives on the road. I put it together with the French thing and thought, if you were going to kill somebody, you'd do it with a motor car accident – it's accepted as an act of God. I wrote a short story that became *The Cars That Ate Paris*. Also over dinner with some friends someone told me of the awful time she had been having with a plumber who had been in her place for a week terrorising her.

Then on a holiday in Tunisia, I found a buried Roman head, a beautiful piece in marble which I somehow knew I was going to find. It was an extraordinary experience. I wondered what it would have been like if a lawyer had found it, someone for whom it was a harder fact to assimilate, the rational man rather than the filmmaker who deals with the imagination. Back in Australia I met the Aboriginal

actor, Gulpilil. I mentioned finding that Roman head and he was
most unimpressed. 'Oh yes,' he said, 'that happens to me all the
time. Of course you know things before they happen.' This became
a starting point for *The Last Wave*. So on that trip to Europe I came
back with what became ideas for three films.

The Cars That Ate Paris

Was it very hard to raise the money for The Cars That Ate Paris,
which had a much bigger budget than Homesdale?
At the time it seemed enormously difficult, but it happened in the
great excitement of the time and it certainly wasn't as difficult as the
experience the producers, Hal and Jim McElroy, had with *Last
Wave* which was very hard to finance, as was *Living
Dangerously*.

That's surprising. The Last Wave *came straight after the success
of* Picnic at Hanging Rock – *I'd have expected finance to be
easy.*
Oh no, you can talk to most filmmakers, you'll find that. You'd
think that for people who win academy awards and make a hundred
million dollars, the next one would be fine. But it's rarely the case –
more often they'll be told 'the last one was excellent, why don't you
do another one like that?' The conservative financial sources tend to
go for what's proven. Mind you, I've always made what I wanted to.
Firstly, I try to keep the budget down and secondly, I only have one
project at a time, unlike the American system where a director will
have five or six going because one of them will go into production
and five won't. I might have five scraps of ideas that I'm turning
over, but only one takes me over.

Cars *was shown at the Melbourne Film Festival, wasn't it?*
Yes. At the end of the picture it was both booed and clapped. That's
been the pattern of my films ever since in one way or another.

You were working with very experienced actors this time.
John Meillon for example. The crew too – they were largely people

who'd worked and been trained on foreign feature films that had been made in Australia. Johnny McLean, who'd been camera operator on *Wake in Fright* was lighting cameraman. Some had worked with Tony Richardson on *Ned Kelly,* or on *Walkabout* with Nick Roeg.

You cast some comic actors from the Melbourne theatre scene. Were you aware of differences in the style of comedy coming from Melbourne and Sydney?
I was aware that in the sixties Melbourne took a different direction; it was far more hard line and political. Sydney is always that rough old seaport, that may take up a trend and play with it; in Melbourne there was far more intensity.

I was struck by the strong kitsch sensibility in Cars, *in the depiction of the Mayor's house and the character of the Mayor's wife.*
Well at that point in my life, I don't know for what reason, I was dealing with the overwhelming normality of things, the ordinariness that sometimes could choke you. And one of the reactions in those days was to satirise. But in *Cars* it was also part of the plot; here was this nice old Mayor and his wife – who looked like anybody's uncle and aunty, with the ticking of the clocks and the tea cosies – and by night these people were killers.

In those early films, parody and satire are an important part of your humour, yet in Gallipoli *the humour is of a very different kind. Why did that change?*
I think I became fond of the people I satirised. The satirist really needs to self-destruct at some point, if he's interested in going further. It's a cul-de-sac and can lead to great bitterness. I had a letter from a friend about *Gallipoli* and he said 'one thing I couldn't get over was the way you treated those characters, those louts in Egypt. As I remember you, you would have satirised them, yet you almost seem to be condoning their actions.' Of course, David Williamson had a great deal to do with the humour in *Gallipoli,* and that was a new and refreshing stimulation for me.

The character of the mayor is rather similar to the manager of the guest house in Homesdale.

It was a constant figure in those early films – the bully, the teacher, the lecturer.

His pretence of concern and sincerity.

It ties in with *Homesdale,* and is very much of that post-Vietnam period. I never took that as far as I wanted to, the feeling of a country in some sort of economic chaos. There were to be troops in the countryside, anarchy in the air, odd radio reports of massive road accidents, politicians being attacked, and so on – there was a whole subplot there. It's interesting when you look at *Mad Max* and *Mad Max 2,* because George Miller said the same thing: that in the first film he got done what he could, but in the second he was able to put in all the texture he'd wanted to in the first.

The grotesque violence and blood in Cars *is also very different from your treatment of violence in* Gallipoli.

Sometimes when you don't know what to do you just make a lot of noise combined with shocking images. There are more subtle things in the film, like the scene after the minister has disappeared and Bruce Spence comes up and just puts his hand in the bloody collar he's wearing and the Mayor looks up. You're constantly trying to hold your audience and it's tempting to lead them with a shock image. But unless it's very carefully arranged, you trigger such strong reactions that you lose the audience for a while. You may want them to do that while something else happens, but generally you get that 'ah' or 'wow' or 'God' and the echoes last up to minutes before they rejoin the picture. And you ask what they thought of the scene and they say 'oh, the scene with the head off' or 'the scene where the lady stands up starkers' and that's all they remember.

Picnic at Hanging Rock

The way the rock is photographed is an important part of Picnic – *how did you decide on all the locations and angles and so on?*

I went down with the executive producer, Pat Lovell, about a year before the film was made and I took photos of the rock. I remember being quite alarmed when I first arrived there that the rock didn't have an impressive distant view. I had expected, with a rock called Hanging Rock, that there would be some fascinating outcrop that gave the place its name. But it didn't look in any sense threatening or particularly powerful and for a long time I planned to do an optical for a wide shot, where I would matte on a further outcrop of rock above the peak, or even move to another location for wide shots. That bothered me for a long time until one morning when we were going to work there was a particular mist across the plain that gave the Rock that element of drama.

Did you shoot that on the spot?
Yes, we stopped all the cars and sent for a camera and anxiously watched the clock as the sun began to heat up the plain and the mist began to rise but we managed to get the shot in.

The artist Martin Sharpe gets a credit on the film – he's called artistic assistant to the director – what was his role?
He was obsessed by the book and had a lot of interesting theories. He came with us to Hanging Rock – we didn't really have a title for him but he was always around the set making suggestions. It was great having him there as somebody to bounce off.

How important are painters and paintings to you in conceiving the look of a film?
I find I gather a folio of prints and photographs before each picture and the walls are covered with them prior to going off to shoot. There can be all sorts of odd things. For example, the whole desert in *Gallipoli* was represented in my own scrapbook by Salvador Dali – those desert landscapes with the huge clocks melting. I always saw Frank and Archie in one of those paintings, walking past one of the clocks.

What about Australian paintings?
I can't recall an image that I carried with me from a particular Australian painting. People often talk of a Tom Roberts influence in *Picnic,* but I wasn't aware of it. I think it's a question of sheer chance – I think I would have as many photographs, postcards, and

advertisements as paintings. They are particularly useful for framing and lighting. Sometimes you collect them and you don't quite know why. But I carry the key ones with me, and sometimes show them to the cameraman in a discussion. I was very interested in *Picnic* in a book of photographs by Lartigue, the French photographer and his early experiments with colour. There's a sort of desaturated look. We did some tests like that, then pulled back from it. I think any time you're dealing with a technique you explore it to its extreme and then attempt to pull away from it, so it's hardly there.

A lot of Picnic *does seem quite muted and softened.*
That was what I wanted. Wendy worked on a monochromatic look. There's something about strong colour in a period film that can disturb. I think it's probably exposure to so many black-and-white photographs.

A lot of people remark on a pre-Raphaelite look about Picnic. *Was that something that you were conscious of at the time in the way you made the girls appear?*
Very much. I knew how they had to look from photographs and paintings. The hard part was finding them. Between Pat Lovell and me, we saw a couple of hundred girls in various States, but by chance we found this particular face, this pre-Raphaelite, nineteenth-century look only in South Australia. You can still see it there – perhaps it's something to do with the way of life. I think of the twenty girls, the large majority were from Adelaide.

It was staggering to see the difference in the girls between Sydney, Melbourne and Adelaide, in one trip. You found in Sydney and Melbourne you had to go younger and younger to find someone who looked right, but that meant other problems. You'd see a fourteen-year-old Sydney girl who might get away with playing a nineteen-year-old nineteenth-century girl, but even then they often looked wrong. It was partly a question of age but more importantly a kind of serenity, or innocence. I think that innocence is in the story and the faces I was drawn to complemented that. Finally, put those faces in that setting, against that rock, and you've got what the book's about.

I've been surprised to hear of classes of schoolgirls today dressing up and going on Picnic at Hanging Rock *picnics: I had the feeling that the film's point of view was that of an outside observer – almost a voyeur – looking at schoolgirls, rather than coming in any way out of a schoolgirl's sense of herself.*

Films viewed at different times and different places can seem very different – shorter, longer, better, worse, didn't ever know it was so funny. This film is obviously viewed very differently now from then, and by schoolgirls with a different view from others. It is a simple and emotive series of images that obviously are still going to touch some people, perhaps young schoolgirls in particular. It is often hard to remember what you intended at the time – the more powerful and ingrained memory is the difficulty you face with each project.

With much of *Picnic at Hanging Rock* it was clearly dangerous ground I was treading on, given the audience's preconditioning, with a mystery that had no solution. I had to supply an ambience so powerful that it would turn the audience's attention from following the steps of the police investigation into another kind of film. I began some technical experiments (which I continued in *The Last Wave*) with camera speeds for example. So within a dialogue scene I would shoot the character talking in the normal 24 frames a second, then I would shoot the character listening in 48 frames, or 32 frames. I would ask the character listening not to blink or make any extreme movement so that you didn't pick up the slow motion, then I'd intercut those reactions and you would get a stillness in the face of the listener. These things were not discernible to the eye, but you would get this feeling, as you sat in your theatre seat, that you were watching something very different.

With the soundtrack I used white noise, or sounds that were inaudible to the human ear, but were constantly there on the track. I've used earthquakes quite a lot, for example, slowed down or sometimes mixed with something else. I've had comments from people on both *Picnic* and *Last Wave* saying that there were odd moments during the film when they felt a strange disassociation from time and place. Those technical tricks contributed to that.

There is a scene during the picnic where Miranda cuts the St Valentine's cake with a huge butcher's knife. Were they things that were added in as you were going or that you conceived in advance?

Most of them were preconceived. It was part of the challenge to switch the audience's expectations, and I was forever looking for things like that knife which would build up a mood where anything was possible. I had to do that as there was so little plot. It was to take the idea of the red herring and to embrace that cliché and pass through it and beyond it, to make so many allusions and connections with images that they were no longer red herrings, but something powerful and unknowable.

The image of the swan that appears towards the end, representing the vanished Miranda, is that from the book?

I think it is – it was pretty outrageous. I was always in two minds about whether to leave it in. I think it's like a lot of things – you make a decision and gamble on it.

The   Last   Wave

The Last Wave *was the film that followed* Picnic. *You've said that the origins of that film lay partly in a conversation with the actor Gulpilil, who plays a lead role in the film.*

Certain scenes in the film were all his, such as those about getting messages from his family through a twitch in his arm – those details were added either by Gulpilil or by Nandjiwara who played Charlie.

How did you find working with Nandjiwara? When you flew up to Darwin to meet him did you find him willing to talk to you about such things?

I spoke initially with Lance Bennett who was director of the Aboriginal Cultural Foundation in Darwin. Obviously you can't just turn up in tribal areas and hope to sit down and talk about a movie. Lance listened to the story, he read the script and we had several meetings before he would even consider it. At first he thought we'd be better off dealing with detribalised people, urban people, but he read further drafts and came to believe that this was a worthwhile project and that there was only one man who could help and that was

Nandjiwara, who is a highly respected tribal elder and magistrate on Groote Island.

So he talked to Nandji about it and showed him the script and after some weeks a meeting was set up. They were actually in Darwin with a dance group from Groote Island, practising prior to leaving for a dance festival in Nigeria. I spent all day with them at Fanny Bay, watching them dance on the beach. I was introduced to Nandji when I arrived. He had a very commanding presence. He indicated that I should come and sit with him and we had tea and smoked cigarettes as his people rehearsed and talked in their language about the rehearsal.

In the first break I turned to him to begin the conversation – I was going to ask what he thought of the script and to expand on it further – and I just looked at that magnificent profile and decided instinctively that I should say nothing at all and left it. That was quite early in the morning and I said nothing all day about it. Then he turned to me at the end of the day and said 'can I bring my wife?' And I knew he was going to do the film. He had been assessing me all day.

I'd brought up a book to show him, a book of Celtic mythology which had struck a chord with me. And he was interested in that. I wanted in the film to show the contrast between the European without the dreaming and the tribal person with the dreaming, and we talked about some of those things. Later, Nandji changed quite a bit of dialogue and asked for certain things to be put in.

Anything that you can remember specifically?
The dinner scene with the family, which is my favourite scene. It is really constructed by Gulpilil and Nandjiwara. Nandjiwara put in all the lines about the law and the law being more important than the man, and that is really the heart of the film. It was a marvellous day's filming, one where you call 'cut' and nothing really changes, the conversation continues. In lunch break they didn't particularly care about leaving, the conversation went on between Richard Chamberlain and Nandjiwara.

What was it like for the white actors and for you as a director working with the Aboriginal actors?

Nandjiwara has such a powerful presence on the set that in a sense
everything came off him when he was working with us. You couldn't
help but be aware of him and one of the points of the film was quite
clearly demonstrated: that very few of us had ever had any contact
with tribal people. There were treasured moments when Nandjiwara
was on the set and one was free to sit with him and have a cup of tea
and talk. It was quite a unique way to meet, given also the heightened
drama and tension of a film set – a sort of no-man's land between
European and Aboriginal. But it was one of those dangerous situations that occur where the making of the film becomes the film, and
that can be an important experience for the film crew, but a lot of it
may not be communicated through the film.

*Did you change much from the written script? How important
was spontaneity in what we see looking at the picture?*
Anything with the Aboriginals underwent change. Nandjiwara was
the key. In accepting to do the film, he accepted the principle of
recreating a lost Sydney tribe and their symbols and tokens. Initially
we made the naive request to use some of his tribal symbols to which
he said absolutely not, nor should we use any existing tribal symbols,
nor should we use any of our collected paintings and drawings of the
vanished Sydney tribe. So Goran Warff, the art director, created a
fictional series of symbols and Nandji approved them.

Nandjiwara had completely grasped this difficult idea, given his
perception of the world, of what 'fiction' is, of what a fiction film is
and how it can give you a truth within its own set of lies. Some of these
concepts were very difficult to get around – the idea of mulkrul, for
instance. It was a word Gulpilil used to describe the other white people
who'd come here before the Europeans; and Nandjiwara had another
word for those people. That was the fascination of this film –
Heyerdahl's theories that the sea is a highway and there have been
many groups and civilizations who have crossed to other countries
and perished or stayed briefly or whatever. And that led me to what I
think was probably too complex in the film: the possibility of a South
American contact, and the idea of mulkrul.

*Because it was your own script were you more open to making
changes than if you were working with something written by*

another person?
Firstly, it was co-written by Tony Morphett. Looking back we should
have gone to another draft because I found myself rewriting it during
the shooting, which is a hellish experience.

It did well in America.
Yes, on the 'art house' circuit. It has its adherents, and there are those
who admire it, particularly in America, much more so than *Picnic*. I
haven't seen it for many years, I haven't been game to look at it.

The   Plumber

The next film you made was the TV movie The Plumber. *Do you
see that as a transition?*
I think it was more a case of saying I could go back to something. *The
Plumber* belonged way back with *Homesdale*. It was done very
quickly and with no fuss, to go straight into television without the
attendant excitement of a cinema release with all its highs and lows. It
reached an audience and played and I thought that's great, I've got
that possibility of working on teleplays.

I have another short story written that I could do in that style at any
time I want to. The change I'd make is to have it on a channel that
didn't have commercial breaks. I would only do it as a complete piece,
or with one interval in the middle. *The Plumber* was made from one
end to the other and played much better that way, given the tension
that built up in the piece and the claustrophobic setting. If I could
control my feature films on television I would. My plan would be to
take a lower fee and hold on to the television rights around the world
and only sell them to people who make one break. But I don't know if
it was any sort of 'transition'.

*I suppose what seems transitional is that while there are
mythical elements, as in your earlier films, you seem much more
distanced from them.*
Well firstly, it was written because I needed the money, which is
sometimes a good way of doing things. It is a true story, though that
is irrelevant to the audience. The couple were friends of mine and the

plumber was based on someone I'd given a lift to once, hitchhiking, and except for the singing in the bathroom and the ending it is pretty much as it happened.

In reality the plumber did leave, but my friend told me, 'the strange thing was that it brought out in me a kind of deviousness, a desire for the survival of my mental state that led me to consider doing really drastic things.' She was an anthropologist, studying those things, so I didn't editorialise. Her story about the incident in New Guinea when the chap came into her room, performed his ceremony or whatever and she tipped milk on him, was all from her thesis. I always thought of recounting that incident as an overture – to indicate that it was all going to happen again.

And she had found herself treating it as some ritualistic thing. Like the fascination with the head of a weaving snake – she really, for her own self-knowledge, had to go through it. She had a certain pride and strength, she was not going to be forced out by this man. And obviously with a situation like that she swung wildly between that and thinking 'I'm going crazy with this whole thing, it is as straightforward as others see it.'

I suppose it seems fairly obvious, but the water motif and the idea of water going beserk is something that has recurred in your films ...
In *Living Dangerously* there was a pool scene and I thought I should cut it out because people had begun to comment on my recurring use of water images. But it's in the book so I went with it. I love working with Ron Taylor who's shot a couple of underwater scenes for me; I'd like to do a film with him sometime, all set under the sea.

Gallipoli

There is an important underwater shot in Gallipoli, *which followed* The Plumber.
That came from the fact that when I first went to Gallipoli I did begin a day down at the beach and swam underwater and was struck by the idea that they had this other particularly peaceful world, where you could float underneath the battlefield so to speak. Down there

nothing had really changed. Then I became intrigued when some old soldier told me about being underwater when they were shelled.

Did you know when you visited Gallipoli that you were going to make the film?
No, but I knew my next film was going to be on the First World War. Probably France. Had it been set in France, it could have been more fictional because so little was known about it, it would have been an entirely different sort of film. The visit changed all of that and I left the peninsula knowing that the film would be about Gallipoli.

Did being there give you a different sense of Gallipoli and what it means for us as Australians?
Not at the time. I was really quite confused by my own emotion there. It took a lot of thinking about. I felt an overwhelming emotion on the evening of the first day and was puzzled about that. I'd had no relatives there, I'd been in battle areas before – I kept thinking it's ridiculous. I think the only comparable feeling I've ever had was at Pompeii which I'd visited back in '65. At Gallipoli, you have an archaeological site really, and it is quite untouched. It's a military zone, no farming and no tourists to speak of because it's so difficult to get to. The war graves are carefully tended, and sited where the men fell.

Are there remnants of the trenches still there?
They are all still there. Now they are only knee deep, but you can wander through the key areas and make your way down Shrapnel Gulley, and you do find a lot of relics there. I brought back a few things. There was a bottle I used in the film and some pieces of shrapnel.

Why do you think Gallipoli has become so important as a theme in Australian culture and ideas?
It was 'the birth of a nation'. Not just the battle and our part in it, but most importantly the referendums on conscription. The troops had landed at Gallipoli in April 1915, and the first referendum on conscription was in 1916. I think that during that twelve months people in Australia had absorbed what had happened over there. It became part of the 'no' vote from the people in the face of the

establishment calling for a 'yes' vote to conscription in this hour of Empire's need. And they were so obviously staggered at the 'no' that they called for the second referendum and got another 'no'. It was the beginning of a turning away from the Empire.

The relationship between the two boys is the central experience of the film – was that emphasis something you got from talking to the returned soldiers?
Yes, given that there are very few first hand accounts. That and the diaries of the soldiers, as compiled by Bill Gammage in a book called *The Broken Years.* It was a way of looking at 'mateship'. When David Williamson and I first looked at it, it seemed a kind of taboo subject, almost too worked over to deal with, but the film became a way of understanding mateship. That's what must have driven us because the drafts became successively less complex as we stripped one element after another out. Earlier drafts dealt with wide aspects of the battle; from Churchill and the meetings of key figures in London, through to the conscription issue.

How important to the concept of mateship is the fact that it's exclusive of women?
Its fundamental. You have to look at the isolation of the outback settlements with women having to cook and have the children, the men going off to work with other men. Mateship came from the bush. Although the bushmen may not have been the majority in the first Australian Imperial Force, Australia's volunteer army, they gave the AIF its flavour. The songs, the poems in The *Bulletin,* and so on were all drawing from their experiences and attitudes. It's often said of male filmmakers that we don't deal effectively with women. I think what's more to the point is that we don't deal effectively with emotion, with feminine aspects of the personality, which are also contained in the male. In a stridently heterosexual, macho society, these are doubly dangerous things to deal with, because they can be easily misconstrued.

Why did you choose to set the early scenes in Western Australia?
In the final attack scene the wave we wanted the boys to go out in was

West Australian. The first two waves went fairly quickly, but that
third wave had that 20, 25 minute wait to see if the attack would
be cancelled. They were West Australian boys and the words of
the officers sending them out was very close to the lines in the
film.

*Why was the desert so important as a setting for part of the lead up
to the departure for Gallipoli?*
It always felt right. At one point we'd planned to intercut the early
outback scenes of Archie with scenes of Frank and his group working
in Perth, contrasting city life with the country. But part of the process
of stripping it down, refining it, was getting Frank out into that
setting. I wanted to give the film that more abstract start – it was an
interesting way to approach a great European war. It also seemed
more truthful, given the importance of the men from the country in
the AIF so I tried to free it from a period feeling to increase that
abstract quality. I kept the costumes to things like khaki shirts,
avoided scenes of city life with cars, horses and carts and so on. In a
sense the 'three acts' of the film took place in three deserts: the
Australian desert, the Egyptian desert, then the desert of Gallipoli –
and over each was that clear blue sky.

The Year of Living Dangerously

Your next film The Year of Living Dangerously, *was set in Asia. For
many people in Australia an interest in Asia and in Eastern ways
of thinking began in the sixties. Was that the case for you too?*
No, not really. On my first trip to Europe in 1965 the first foreign port
was Colombo. I only spent a day there but it did have a great impact on
me. My interest has increased with the years, and further travels.

How did you make the decision to make The Year of Living
Dangerously?
I don't know – you're going back to a choice made in 1978, prior to
doing *Gallipoli,* when I took the rights out. So it's always a curious
thing that you make a choice to do something on a certain inspiration
at a time, then you find you're dealing with it two or three years later,

with certain changes of perspective. I was excited by the book, that was the starting point.

One of the most interesting aspects of The Year of Living Dangerously *is that it is set very much in an Asian context and yet the sensibility of Billy Kwan, which is so central to the film, is essentially a Christian sensibility. Do you identify with his attitudes?*

Only some of them – I think that's what I found interesting about the character. I've certainly softened him rather – I think he was less likeable in the novel. What I did like about Billy was his talk about the wayang, the Indonesian shadow puppet plays, and its possibilities. I felt Billy finally perishes because he gives up his own belief in the wayang. It was the Eastern aspects I was drawn to, not the Western, but they are in opposition and that is part of the story. I just altered the balance in the mix. And Linda Hunt, who played Billy, altered it further.

Making the Chinese-Australian dwarf, Billy Kwan, an androgynous sort of character represents a real change from Christopher Koch's book where I gather he is a much more unequivocally masculine figure.

I needed to equal the originality of Koch's creation in the novel. It was an accident or rather sheer desperation that led me to Linda though now it seems to form a sort of pattern. I was dealing with an almost mythical character – something like a Grimm's fairy tale character who had been transformed by a witch into a hunchback, or a frog. Then of course, there's Beauty and the Beast and Quasimodo. I had to ask myself how important was the question of height, because on screen, close up, the height difference would be far less perceptible, so even casting a very short man (which had proved very difficult) would not capture the feeling I needed. I needed something more. I did at one stage contemplate putting a hunchback onto the character, going much further in a grotesque physical way to make him a prisoner of the body. I got very excited when I began to think of the incredible implications of casting Linda. So I built the film around that and embraced that casting. A risky decision, but it paid off.

Certainly many people who don't know that Linda Hunt is a woman read the character as a man.

I've had all the reactions and they all seem to join up to the same point: finally it doesn't matter. Her performance is what matters.

The image of the wayang is carried through in the love story and the interaction between the characters. How happy do you feel with the translation of that imagery in the political sphere. Were you trying to develop it in the same way?

It was an interesting background for me. There was a glimpse of a dictator who had begun with all the best intentions, and a quick sketch of a patriot, Kumar, giving another angle on 'communist' which is such an emotive word. But they were quick sketches, they didn't really interest me terribly. I wanted a rather timeless setting in that background. The film was about Asia to me, and the background was to reflect that. I always felt that if you didn't know anything about it, it wouldn't matter. But I don't think you are ever truly happy with a finished film. It was a complex adaptation and over a dozen drafts David Williamson and I were constantly altering the balance of the elements. I think there is enough of the political story there, but you often have to look into the frame to find it.

So the specifics of the coup in Indonesia were not of primary concern for you?

They gave rise to certain attitudes and reactions from the characters, as with *Gallipoli*.

You were asked some years ago about the similarity between your work and Nicholas Roeg's and you observed that Roeg uses sexuality as part of the tension in his films where you use other systems. But in Living Dangerously *you decided to deal with sex directly.*

It was part of the story; it was simply appropriate to use it. I was quite interested to take it on as it was my first attempt at that kind of relationship. I think it is probably there in my earlier work – there is obviously a sexual tension in *Picnic at Hanging Rock*.

The character of Guy Hamilton in The Year of Living Dangerously *makes a decision that is fairly unconventional in movie terms in that he chooses to join Jill Bryant and leave Indonesia, abandoning the chance of reporting the biggest story of his career. The character of Jill Bryant herself is fairly unconventional – less passive and mindless than many female film roles.*

I made some quite major changes from the character in the novel – I didn't see the Jill of the novel, I didn't like her. And so I worked with Sigourney Weaver on constructing a woman that we found interesting – a combination of strength and femininity.

In the book she is pregnant when she gets on the plane. It makes a very big difference that she is not pregnant in the film.

I thought it would be dangerous in a movie: I don't know how one would ever separate guilt from desire in the action of Hamilton in joining her. It is desire not just for her, but to rejoin his own personality. He is like a man who has lost his shadow towards the end; the only way he can ever continue to be a good journalist and a complete human being is to take that plane. It was one of those significant choices, which Hamilton might have found hard to explain to people, those who could not comprehend his leaving the job. It is in those lines of Kwan's: 'why can't you give yourself; why can't you open yourself up; why can't you learn to love?' They are from the novel and they seem to me to be true.

The filming of the last sequence seems to get a mixed reaction from people who watch it. Had you always had that ending in mind?
Yes. It never changed. I always knew it was unfashionable.

Mel Gisbon's walk across the tarmac . . .
One of my favourite moments in the film is the mid-shot of Mel as he crosses the tarmac. We did several takes and I think the only thing I asked him to do was to smile, which was the only major development in the scene. I said 'I can't describe it, but there's a special smile, a kind of release. Not from getting out of customs, but in a sense of rejoining yourself; it's like two images that come together.' And he did that thing of tipping his head back . . . and to me the film was over.

It's what the film has been about. I realise that some people don't
follow the clues through from the beginning and the danger is that if
you expect the film to conform to a traditional genre or to one's own
view of life and people, then all the earlier fragile elements will be
missed and the result will be confusing. Some of the more didactic
critics asked in their reviews 'what kind of film *is* this – is it a love
story, is it a thriller, is it a political story?' You could say that it
unsuccessfully fails to fuse these elements, but to ask why deal with
all those elements together, why not choose one of them, reveals a
view of life and films that is very different from my own.

Some said 'oh yes, here we have the old moral malaise of the
Westerner, the dilemmas from the sixties that we're all so familiar
with.' But I'm sorry, these issues don't just go away – we don't stop
wondering about the enormous gap between the Third World and our
world; we don't stop thinking about love, or about how to construct
some sort of moral system, and all those elements are touched on within the film. Most of my films have been left incomplete, with the viewer
as the final participant: I don't like the didactic approach. One is constantly left wondering and I love it when that's done to me in a film.

R E F L E C T I N G   O N   D I R E C T I N G

W a t c h i n g   M o v i e s

How do you want your films to affect people?
I like to think that people get their money's worth, that I've
entertained them, because I belong to that tradition of entertainer or
storyteller. There's this cartoon up on my wall of an old lady at a ticket
box window saying 'I want my sense of wonder back.' I like that idea.
It's a desire to feel that sense of not knowing, that sense of danger and
potential interlocked. It's very difficult to achieve, but the screen is
one of the few places where it is possible.

Do you enjoy going to the movies?
Very much, yes. But I'm very selective, very careful – if I see a film I
really don't like it depresses me . . . in the sense of what a waste of time

this whole occupation is. I tend to watch them at home, because you can take them off. I don't have a video because I don't like the format as much as I do the screen, but I have my own 16mm setup and I borrow from the libraries and film exchanges. It seems to go in bursts – I might have an 'on' period when I watch dozens of movies, then nothing for weeks or months.

Are there filmmakers who have been particularly influential for you?
I didn't really investigate any film history up until 1978. I was making *The Plumber* in Adelaide for the South Australian Film Corporation, they have an excellent film library there and I used to watch four or five features a week – I put myself through a film history course.
The emphasis was heavily on silent films and many of them just took my breath away. Of the early Russian filmmakers I came to admire Pudovkin, to my surprise. I thought it would be Eisenstein, but although I appreciated his intellect, I found him too much a propagandist. I liked the naive, almost primitive approach of Pudovkin, and his passion and emotion. I couldn't do anything but admire the lighting and composition of the Germans, but they didn't move me greatly. I loved Hitchcock's films, his wit, his effortless quality. In the commercial cinema it was Kubrick who had an enormous effect on me. I would go to the Sydney Film Festival, and I was interested in European cinema. And Kurosawa, I still carry around images from his films.
   But I'm not aware of any direct influence, perhaps because I am a little like a primitive painter myself – you know, those painters whose trees are a little too big or whose cows only stand sideways, and who paint out of sheer joy and intuitive understanding. I have been aware of the dangers of refining the craft and losing the art. In latter years I have been inspired by Woody Allen – I admire his recklessness. He's an original and that is true of all the filmmakers I have mentioned. I've turned away from the more academic filmmakers, or the social workers. Godard reminded me of that university lecturer who had demolished the Blake poem.

Are there any of your own films you don't like later?
Yes. Although when I say dislike, that's excepting certain scenes.

Then there are others that at the time you thought were less successful, but seem to age well. It's a curious pattern.

Working on the Set: Democracy and Intuition

Do you consciously do things to engender an atmosphere on a set? Do you have established approaches at the start of a film?
I think it just happens. An extraordinary feeling of the proximity of chaos hovers around a film set. That is dangerous to the director because it is all-pervasive and you can get very rattled. People are under great stress and are very excited and determined to do their best. I presume it's true on every set: the feeling that you have been selected for this position and that you're going to have to prove your worth. And in the early days of a shoot people trip and knock things over – the old jokes about people on the set bumping into lamp-stands are literally true – until the unit is in rhythm, which sometimes doesn't happen until quite late. Then everything settles down, but in those early weeks it can be very chaotic and you need to develop your own approach to combat that, to harness it, or your ideas can begin to disintegrate.

Is your approach to directing actors in comedy very different from directing drama?
It's the same thing really. I build an atmosphere on the set that is conducive to the performing of the scene. The script to me is only a starting point. Coming from a tradition of ad-libbing and improvising, I need that atmosphere. So I try to keep the equipment to a minimum, and to keep it out of the way of the actors. It's a case of creating a powerful mood, a kind of 'super-reality' out of which the actors' responses will be both irresistable and inevitable, be it comedy or drama.

Shooting on location must make a difference to the atmosphere of the film, as opposed to being in a town.
If the weather's good and the period is not too extended it can be wonderful. For example during the week that we shot all the outback

scenes for *Gallipoli* we were in a caravan city attached to an old cattle station. The weather was perfect: hot during the day and crisp and cool in the evening. We had log fires and people told yarns or sang songs. With *Picnic* we started off in Mount Macedon where we were billeted in various old guest houses. It was a beautiful area – it was idyllic. On the other hand shooting in Manila, where we were on location with *Living Dangerously,* was very arduous.

Francis O'Brien, the American executive producer on Gallipoli, *commented on the degree of democracy in that production, and as a general characteristic of the Australian film industry as opposed to the American. Is that something you're aware of?*
I'm sure its cultural. In Britain, and to a degree in America, they do call the director 'sir', and some of the older Australian crew members who'd gone through foreign features here used to call me 'sir' in the early days, to my amazement. I said 'don't worry about that' at one stage, but then I realised that's as much an affectation as wearing a baseball cap, in the Australian context. In America it's very highly competitive, people have really fought their way up and won the right to be in the position of assistant director or cameraman or whatever, and there can be a much larger degree of compartmentalising, and respect for those above you. And a keen awareness that you can be fired, which is much more the American way.

That's not been the case in Australia. Obviously we couldn't do it, we've had to inspire each other – in the seventies there was one of everybody. We were all learning together in those early days, so you were pooling knowledge, with that one common desire to make the picture look as good as anything from anywhere else. But more importantly it's probably just part of our way of doing things – you can see it in the army during the war; there was much more negotiation between officers and men in the Australian forces than in the British.

Do you prefer in general to be completely prepared before you go onto the set? The Last Wave *sounds like an example of considerable spontaniety.*
That was true of that film, but generally I don't like that way of doing things. I did in my early days but I've simply found it too difficult – you run the risk of losing control.

When threats were made by a Muslim extremist group during the shooting of The Year of Living Dangerously *in the Philippines, you moved the shoot back to Australia, saying 'life first, movie second'. Earlier you might have been tempted to stay and explore the possibilities created by that tension.*

I prefer it that way, as did most of the cast and crew. Filmmaking is a craft for me. I like the approach of the Japanese master potter who turns each bowl out one after the other, the last exactly the same as the first. Occasionally the gods descend and touch his hands as he makes one of those bowls and that one is inspired, a work of art. The danger of 'movies first, life second', is the danger of the filmmaker as god. So I have been drawn away from that toward the craft aspect, leaving these other things to chance. And I don't think you necessarily lose anything, that's the interesting discovery.

C o n s t r u c t i n g   t h e   P i c t u r e s

The relationship between the director and director of photography seems to be a very key one. You've worked a lot with Russell Boyd – have you developed a special way of working together?

Yes. Of course, until *Living Dangerously* there was also Johnny Seale who was a very important part of the camera team as camera operator. He is now working as a director of photography. So it was really very much Russell Boyd, John Seale, myself, and Wendy Weir. Few people realise when you talk about the lighting of a picture you must also talk about what light is falling on. Here two important aspects come into play: firstly, and most importantly, it's the faces that are being photographed, whether extras or key cast; and secondly, the settings into which they are placed. That team interlocked very well. Russell would light those faces very well, would repsond to the faces and the setting, and John Seale would move the camera beautifully amongst and through and around them. Wendy has looked after colour on all those pictures. Not only the colour of the sets and the costumes but the key colours of the film – in *Gallipoli* for example, you have sand, khaki, and blue.

And Russell is absolutely superb in exterior situations. You'll find a

number of cameramen who are very good with candlelit ambience in a
room, but there are very few people who can use a landscape well. To
work in the middle of the day in Australia where you've got that harsh
overhead sun which is a very unflattering light and to turn it
somehow to advantage takes real skill. In the films that we've done
together, I think particularly of the actual picnic in *Picnic at
Hanging Rock*. That was done over a period of a week for one hour
only, I think between twelve and one, when Russell found the light
was at its most interesting. He scrimmed a parachute silk or
something above them to soften the light. The techniques are well
known but the difference is that it took, with a very low budget, an
enormous amount of clever juggling of the schedule and Russ's
insistence that we shoot only at that hour to capture that look which
became a key element of the film. And also, I think of his
photographic work in the scenes of the boys crossing the desert in
Gallipoli, and the way he used the light in those sequences.

*Where are the decisions about the composition and framing of a
shot made? Do you look through the camera much yourself?*
It depends on the operator. When you build up a strong rapport as I
did with Johnny Seale – we worked together on *Picnic, Last Wave*
and *Gallipoli* – you don't need to look very often. I don't do a story
board because for me a lot of the pages are blank. There are sequences
which I know must look a particular way, and those ones are easy: I'd
say 'I want to do it this way' and Johnny would look through and
improve it. But with scenes that were unplanned, I'd throw myself
into the rehearsal and Johnny would watch closely and then I'd turn
to him and say 'what do you think of that? Did you see her when she
turned?' and he'd have got all those things.

So, in other words, the ideas would come from me but the framing
and realisation were often John's. I was constantly impressed with the
way that he would take that idea, and with a different framing, he
would come up with a new idea. And given that as a director you want
to conserve energy and throw yourself into breaches in the wall, so to
speak, I could leave a lot of the framing and movement to John.

Music, Philosophy, Success

You've mentioned the importance of music. I take it you weren't talking about music on the soundtrack, but about music as a source for you?
An inspiration really. I have a fantastic collection of tapes, of many different kinds of music. I'll find that I play half a dozen tapes constantly during the writing period. Sometimes they find their way into the film, because I realise that I directed the scene with the music in mind. That happened with the piece of Vangelis in *Living Dangerously*. Maurice Jarre was booked to do the music, but I'd loved this piece from an early Vangelis album and I used it in two places – the scene where they drive through the roadblock and later where Sigourney Weaver comes up the steps to Mel Gibson at his office.

You will actually play music on the set while a scene is shot?
Quite often. Though I think it's only a last resort during the actual shooting. And I'll only do it if I know that the music won't disturb the cast, otherwise I'd be imposing a mood on them which might inhibit their performance. But it's a way of blocking out the creak of the camera dolly, the ping of insects on the lights, or the sound of distant laughter from outside the studio. It's a way of detaching them, and me, from the dozens of pairs of eyes that are watching, and it helps me to fight back the overwhelming weight of ordinariness that surrounds you in daily life, to recall the inspiration. For some actors, of course, it's of no particular interest. Mel Gibson, for example, finds it curious that I play odd bits of music, but it's not his music and he's not particularly interested – he doesn't need it and I keep it away from him.

There has been a continuing current of interest in mysticism in your films. Are you attracted to any major thinkers or groups?
I react against the organised aspects of 'spiritual' studies, which is probably a better word. Writers who interest me are those who span several disciplines: Carl Jung has probably been the most important for me. To Jung I'd add Thor Heyerdahl, and Emmanuel Velikovsky with his books *Worlds in Collision* and *Ages in Chaos* where he

puts together theories using elements of archaeology, astrology, geology, and biology. But any of these writers, Freud as well of course, have been ostracised and condemned by the leaders of individual disciplines. That spanning of so many disciplines and possibilities seems to me to be particularly applicable to films. Yet tragically even in its brief history, film is becoming formalised and institutionalised by academics.

How do you measure the success of a film for yourself? How important is it that a film does well at the box office?
In the end I look back to see how close I've come to capturing the original inspiration. The percentage of success varies from film to film. As for the box office, it's like they say – luck and timing.

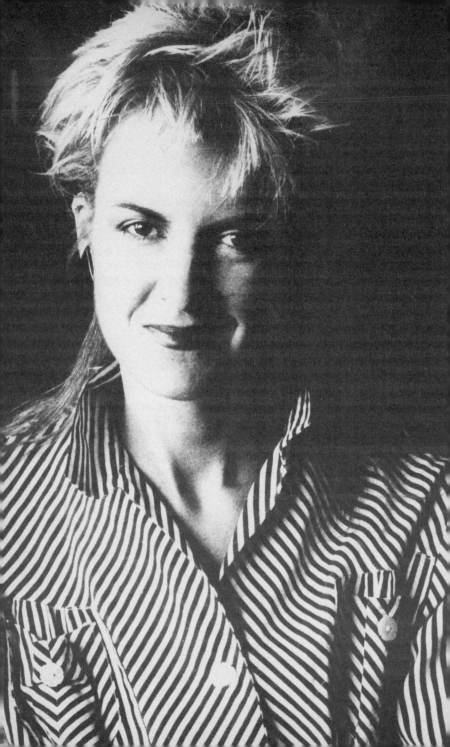

GILLIAN ARMSTRONG

Gillian Armstrong belongs to what she calls the 'second generation' of current Australian filmmakers. During the adolescence and early working lives of directors like Fred Schepisi and Peter Weir, the pursuit of a career as a film director was regarded as an ambition at best fanciful, at worst bizarre and irresponsible. But when Armstrong moved from high school to college in 1968, she found herself at the Melbourne home of the first practical film training course in Australia, the Swinburne Institute of Technology. The ambition to become a fully fledged feature-film director took some time to emerge, but its hatching coincided with the opening of the Sydney-based national Australian Film and Television School and Armstrong was among the first class in the directors' course at 'the Film School'.

Armstrong is in the rather unusual position of having experienced the early days of the cinema revival in both Melbourne and Sydney. By the time she graduated from the Film School, the film renaissance was solidly in progress: she explains how for her the system of government grants for filmmakers was so taken-for-granted that she only became aware of the unique possibilities it offered after meeting young filmmakers overseas who lacked such advantages.

With the aid of a grant she made the fifty-minute *The Singer and the Dancer* (1976), acting as producer as well as director and co-writer. Then in 1977 producer Margaret Fink enlisted her to direct *My Brilliant Career,* based on the nineteenth-century novel by Australian writer Miles Franklin. It was a bold move: the decision to use not just a director who had never made a feature film, but a young, female director who had never made a feature film raised a lot of eyebrows in the Australian film industry in 1977. It was a time when awareness of the systematic bias against women was beginning to open some previously all-male doors, and indeed the Australian film industry employs a higher proportion of women than many others. Still, contemporary Australia is not known for pioneering the advance of feminism and it was a doubly significant achievement when *My Brilliant Career* became one of the major films in Australia in 1979. Though the film has been criticised as being insufficiently biting or challenging, those very qualities may well have contributed to its appeal. It was well received at the Cannes Film Festival and, with Bruce Beresford's *Breaker Morant, My Brilliant Career* led the penetration of the American market by Australian films, becoming a favourite with American 'art house' audiences. *My Brilliant Career* established Gillian Armstrong as one of Australia's leading directors. It did the same for Judy Davis, establishing her as one of the leading film actors in Australia.

Armstrong's second feature, *Starstruck* (1982), was a contemporary pop musical. Despite the razzle dazzle with which it was launched the film met with a fairly tepid response in Australia; American critics and audiences have been kinder. *Starstruck* enabled Armstrong to make use of her continuing interest in youth culture and fashion. She had initially planned to be a theatre designer, and worked as art director on a number of feature films. From her student films on, visual flair and a strong concern for the appearance of things have characterised all Armstrong's films. An interest in style is evident even in the way Gillian Armstrong looks herself: her dress is studied, yet casual and idiosyncratic.

The peculiar status of being one of the few successful women directors of feature films – and the only one, so far, in Australia – is something of which Armstrong is very conscious. She talks with some fervour of the difficulties that have confronted her, and that challenge all women working in films. She does not identify herself with the organised women's movement, but the lives of women and the effects on them of their social circumstances are a major focus in her work. In 1977 she directed a sensitive documentary called *Smokes and Lollies*, about the lives of three fourteen-year-old, working-class girls. Four years later she went back to make a follow-up about the same girls, called *Fourteen's Good, Eighteen's Better*. She is anxious not to be typecast as a director of 'women's films', though she has found herself drawn to stories about women. It's indicative that when asked who are the actors she particularly

admires, Armstrong immediately names women, the male actors
occuring to her only secondarily.

That women in their professional capacity are treated differently
from men in the film industry (as in most places) was demonstrated in
the course of conducting the interview with Armstrong. She talked
far more frankly about the pressure the work of a film director places
on her personal life than any of the male directors had done. It was
possible to pursue those questions with her in a way that seemed
much more difficult with the male directors: questions that are
regarded by both interviewer and interviewee as appropriate, even
predictable in talking to a woman are often seen as 'intrusive' or
'irrelevant' in interviews with men. None of us, it seems, have
progressed quite as far as we'd like to think.

One of the actors Armstrong mentioned was Diane Keaton and in
fact her current project is a film to be financed by MGM and made in
America in which Keaton will star with Australian Mel Gibson. 'I
didn't think it would happen so fast,' says Armstrong, who at the time
of this interview indicated only that she 'might' go to the US if she
found a script she liked enough. She is ensuring a degree of
continuity with her Australian work by taking with her not only a
cinematographer (Russell Boyd), but also a designer (Luciana
Arrighi) and an editor (Nick Beauman).

Asked where her family came from originally Armstrong replies,
'Scotland – can't you tell? Armstrong: we even have our own tartan.
I'm the original Anglo-Australian, Scottish and English on both
sides.' Her grandfather was mayor of Nunawading, an outer suburb
of Melbourne and she grew up in nearby Vermont, where her father,
an enthusiastic amateur photographer, took over the family
real-estate business. Her grandmother, she says, remembers when
there were Aboriginal camps on the nearby hills; by 1950, though,
when Gillian was born, the surburban sprawl had spread to Vermont
and the replacement of the old orchards by brick veneer villas was well
and truly underway.

Despite an initial reluctance to undertake this interview, Gillian
Armstrong proved very forthcoming, and very generous with her
time. She is an amusing conversationalist, with a quick, staccato
delivery. A slightly scatty, throwaway style covers a thoughtful and
clearly an effective personality. She makes frequent ironic asides and

often illustrates her answers with self-deprecating anecdotes. Yet she has a reputation for being strong-willed, even dictatorial, on the set, and brooking little disagreement. The apparent contradiction between those two modes seems characteristic. She is clearly confident and assured about her self and her ability, yet her reluctance to be interviewed – 'because I haven't done anything yet that is really worth talking about' – accompanies a genuine acknowledgement of flaws in her films and of what remains to be learned.

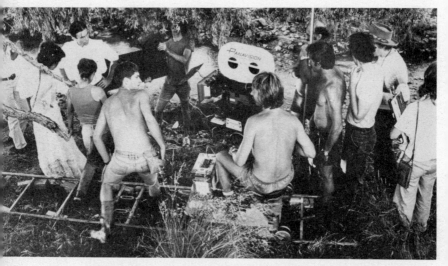

Above: Intimacy by the river in *My Brilliant Career*. The director has her back to the camera, talking to the actors Judy Davis and Sam Neill in the left of the shot.

Above right: 'There was a sudden interest in Australian icons . . . I think it's great, but at the moment I feel like if I see another Sydney t-shirt, I'll scream.' Ross O'Donovan (Angus Mullens), in kangaroo suit, and Jo Kennedy (Jackie Mullens) arrive at the rock club in *Starstruck*.

Below right: 'I thought I should do a youth film before I got too old.' Jo Kennedy (Jackie Mullens) and dancers on stage with The Swingers, led by Phil Judd, in the Sydney Opera House climax of *Starstruck*.

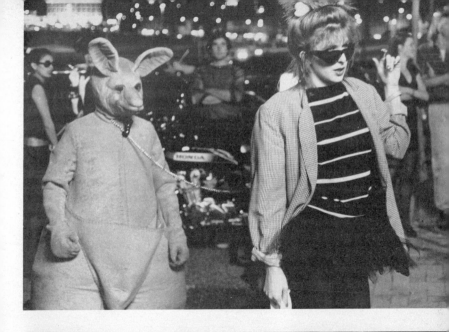
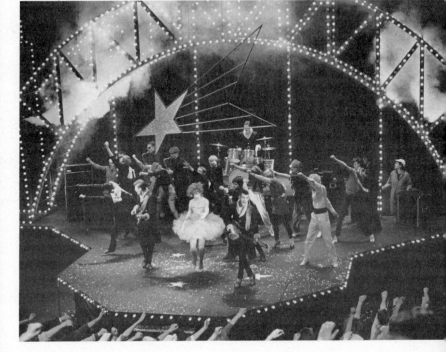

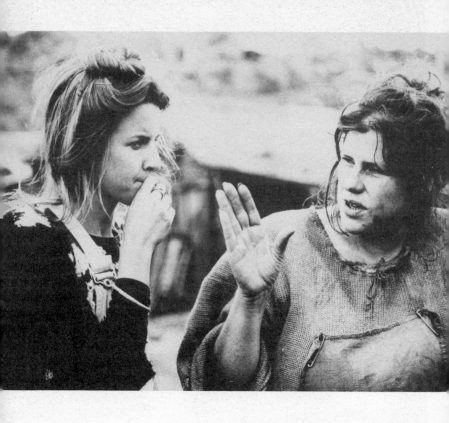

Above: Gillian Armstrong and Carole Skinner (Mrs McSwat) on the set of *My Brilliant Career.*

Right: Sam Neill (Harry Beecham), Judy Davis (Sybylla Melvin) and Gillian Armstrong on the set of *My Brilliant Career.*

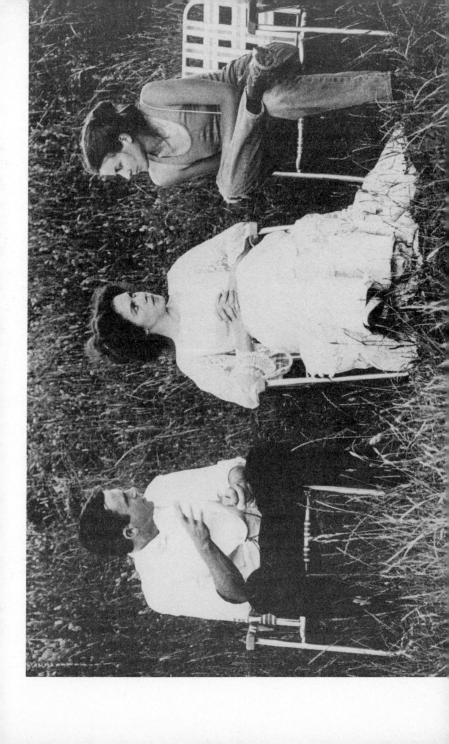

BEGINNINGS

A Hybrid Cultural Childhood

Sue Mathews: Many of the current generation of filmmakers in Australia – Phillip Adams, Peter Weir, Bruce Beresford – talk about how important the Saturday afternoon matinées were for them, but you probably just missed that whole Saturday arvo matinée culture. Did you go to the movies much as a kid?

Gillian Armstrong: No, not really – I was part of the television generation. Television came to Melbourne in 1956 with the Olympic Games, when I was six. The man next door owned an electrical store, so he was the first in the neighbourhood to have a TV set, and we all used to climb over the fence and go and sit in giant groups around the TV. I did see a few children's sessions of Saturday matinées, but there were no real cinemas in the outer suburbs, and it was three quarters of an hour by train to the city.

What sorts of things did you do?

It seems so pretentious talking about your childhood ... I used to write my own plays, and my sister and I would make costumes and organise performances in the garage with all the kids. I was an obsessive bookworm too; I used to put the light under the blankets and keep reading hours after I was meant to.

A lot of the children's literature available then seemed to come from England.

Yes, they were generally English books, like *The Secret Garden* by Frances Hodgson Burnett. When I was going through the primary school system there was a great push about being Australian and reading Australian literature, but I hated all that stuff – Henry Lawson's *The Loaded Dog,* things like that. It was about deserts, goldminers and bushrangers and things that were not part of my life. Even so, England always seemed very far away. But it's an interesting dichotomy in Australia – on one hand most of the children's books I read were English and yet all the early TV was American. I liked *Leave it to Beaver, Shirley Temple's*

Wonderland and *Disneyland*. Oh, and Ricky Nelson in *Ozzie and Harriet*. I quite fancied Ricky. But it's funny seeing the replays, because I see that he's about nine and I think, was I fancying boys then? I must have been about eight.

Did that American life that was presented on TV seem as far away from you as the English life that you read about in books?
Well I sure understood that they both weren't here. But I preferred the English TV programs. European-based things have always seemed richer to me. It was the boys who got into the Americana. I actually used to hate cowboys and Indians – I remember whenever the Indians attacked the wagon train I had to be carried out screaming. But generally I had the feeling that American programs were trashy. I don't know how early that was developed.

It's interesting – the previous generation thought the Americans were wonderful; they saved us in the war, and the soldiers on R & R were so glamorous in World War Two.
I know I grew up to be quite anti-American. That was reinforced in the seventies, because of Vietnam and so on. But it was so much part of me – I used to say that I couldn't stand talking to a person with an American accent, they used to irritate me.

The exception to that was movies on TV – I've always been an addict of American cinema of the thirties and forties, which was generally shown as the midday movie. At high school I had a friend who lived next door to the school so we used to sneak over the fence at lunchtime to watch the old Humphrey Bogart and Bette Davis movies, and if it was a good one we'd miss the first period after lunch. Also being the least valued person on any sports team, I had even greater impetus to escape.

Was pop music important to you?
Yes, I've always been really involved – as a fan – with rock music. The Beatles started happening just at the age when I first became interested in music. I forgot to mention earlier that one of the TV shows I used to rush home from school for was *Kommotion,* the great mime program. And because I lived out near the Channel 0

studios, where the weekly rock program *The Go Show* was produced, I used to go regularly and watch. And at that stage I think I'd already decided that I wanted to do something in TV or film, because I used to tell my family that I wasn't just going to look at Billy Thorpe and the Easybeats and Normie Rowe – I'd come home and talk about all the sets being done in tones of blue and things.

So you had decided at an early age you were interested in working in film or television?
Yes, or design. When I was eleven one of my teachers told my mother that I had some talent as an actress – I used to give myself star roles in a lot of my plays – so I started taking speech and drama lessons from Miss Daphne Powell at the Mitcham memorial hall every Wednesday afternoon. I did that for almost seven years. At school I was always a very conscientious student but by fifth form I was sick of studying and I decided to do General Art at Swinburne technical college.

Film School Number One: Swinburne

Was the film course at Swinburne already going then?
It had been going for about four years at that stage. The original lecturers were mostly graphic artists who had got interested in film. In fact the course started because one of the staff, Brian Robinson, wanted to make a movie and talked the education department into buying some equipment. It was the first film course in the country. But originally, because I was very much caught up in youth culture, I thought I'd either be a theatre designer or a fashion designer. Then during my first year I saw some student films – that was the first time film seemed accessible to me in any sense. Besides, all the third and fourth year boys looked so spunky running around in the back alleys with their faces painted white. I think I probably liked the idea of making these arty little films, with people running around lanes.

When did you develop a major interest in feature films?
It was through Swinburne. In second year we started to study film

history and film theory. Every Tuesday morning Jim Harris – I think he's still there – used to show us the great classics. We saw hundreds of films. At the beginning of that year we were asked to name our favourite film. I'm sure I put down *The Graduate,* but there was someone next to me who put down *Wild Strawberries* by Bergman, and I was wondering 'who's this Bergman?' Then, 'who's this Griffith? Who's this Eisenstein?' I mean, it just hadn't been part of my world at all. The films I was most attracted to at that stage were films like de Sica's *Bicycle Thieves* and a lot of early Italian and French cinema – I liked the strength of the images and the feeling and of course I was touched by the human stories and the social content of a lot of those early black-and-white films. I'd never seen anything like them: they don't get out to the suburbs.

And what about American movies – had you been going to commercial cinema much?
Well, American films were sort of frowned on. Once you get into art school you become a great cultural snob. That's one thing you're taught very early on – it's like me being embarrassed about writing down *The Graduate.* As a teenager I did go to the movies – I can remember going to see the Gerry and the Pacemakers film *Ferry Across the Mersey* and forcing my mother to take me to see *Georgie Girl.*

They're both English films, interestingly enough.
I was a mod, you see! I mean, in the sixties, the music was English, the fashion was English, everything good seemed to be English. There was Mary Quant and The Stones and The Who and all that, and everybody who could used to go straight to London. But with this cultural snobbishness of mine, I even refused to go and see *Bonnie and Clyde.* I used to say that I wouldn't be manipulated by the media. I thought if they could afford to put a full page ad for their film in the newspaper, I wouldn't go and see it.

Did you do much actual production at Swinburne? Did you get to run around in back lanes?
Yes, lots of that. Swinburne was a very, very poor film school and I realise now that the idea was to stall us actually running film through

the camera because it cost so much. In the first year we did animation, which is very clever because you're shooting it frame by frame so you spend six months on one hundred feet. For editing exercises, we used offcuts from Crawford's, who made all the TV cop shows. We had books that said 'this person looks to the left and this one looks to the right and when you cut them together they'll be looking at each other.' For me it was just like a foreign language.

Were you involved with people outside Swinburne who were trying to make films? Fred Schepisi mentioned that you had done some work on his segment of Libido.
Nigel Buesst was a lecturer and he was a *real* filmmaker. He was part of the Carlton scene, where people were making independent films, and he tried to establish some sort of contact for Swinburne with the industry. Fred Schepisi also used to visit as an assessor – he's always been very generous with his time with young filmmakers, and he'd given a lot of very talented people a break at The Film House. Ian Baker, who shot all Fred's films, was a Swinburne graduate. Fred had liked my little graduation film, *The Roof Needs Mowing* and they offered me a job doing continuity on *Libido*. I was out of town when they rang and missed out on the job offer, but they still said 'why don't you just come along for the experience.' So I was actually tea girl on *Libido*. That was shot in December 1971 when I was 21 – it was wonderful. Fred is still the most inspiring director I've ever seen at work, he has power with people that I feel I'll never match.

The   Cultural   Cringe

How were the first of the new Australian films received?
I remember going to see Tim Burstall's *2000 Weeks,* during its two-day run in Melbourne in 1969, and what a shock it was to hear an Australian accent on the screen, how funny it sounded, and not quite right. I think *Picnic at Hanging Rock* was the film that first affected Australian audiences. People felt 'we don't have to be embarrassed anymore.' That's why it was so hyped: people felt 'here's a film that's beautiful and it's real', and suddenly Australian accents were forgiven.

Was that really the first Australian film to be accepted – what about the ocker comedies that had come before Picnic?

I think it was the first real breakthrough. *Alvin Purple* did make a lot of money and was a very popular film and so were the *Barry McKenzie* films, but I think the new middle-class cinema audience still regarded them as not particularly worthwhile, as a bit cheap and nasty. We probably needed one serious film before we could laugh at ourselves as well. I think it was still the old cultural cringe: 'this is not the way we want the English to see us.' We wanted to show them that we were just as sophisticated as they were and that we read books too. The audience's familiarity with Australian material through the growing success of TV soaps made a difference too.

Why do you think the ocker comedies made up such a large proportion of the early seventies films?

Well, I remember reading Tim Burstall's letters to the press over the years. *2000 Weeks* was made as a very serious film and it was savagely attacked by the critics. Obviously he was very hurt, and I do think he was unfairly savaged, because while there were serious flaws in the film, its intentions were very honourable. But in Australia we really do come down on ourselves. It's almost like we don't really believe that we can do it and every time anyone tries something that fails they're really roasted by the press. It's like, 'there, see, we couldn't do it' and 'look at how dreadful it is.' It's almost as if the press feel it's themselves up there being exposed and that's why they attack it so strongly.

So Tim Burstall came out and said things like 'the public doesn't want art and I'm not going to make it anymore – it's more important to bring the message to a wider audience than to an elite and so I'm going to make commercial films.' He made the *Alvin Purple* films, *Stork, Petersen,* a lot of those early ones. I think the press really had an effect on him as a filmmaker. Although I do think that *Stork* manages to do both successfully.

Down   and   Out   in   Sydney

Did you move to Sydney with a clear intention of getting into the film industry?
Well, yes. It seemed that the only places to go in Melbourne were the commercial film houses – a lot of Swinburne students went into advertising or Crawfords, the cop show producers. Film Australia, which used to be the Commonwealth Film Unit, where Peter Weir started, just used to put my letters on file, and when I wrote to the ABC they wrote back asking me my typing speed – they didn't even want to look at my films.

So I had a rude awakening: after five months of waitressing I realised that it might even be quite stimulating to work in a commercial film house – anything rather than clear people's plates away. It was fun to be in exciting Sydney, and getting on the ferries and going back and forth across the harbour, but I started to get worried that I'd never get my foot in the door. I think I grew up a lot in that time.

The best advice I was ever given was from the people at *Spyforce*, where they couldn't give me a job but advised me to go into editing. I'd still thought 'well, a girl does continuity' so that was what I should do. It was lucky because I was always really hopeless at organizing with stop watches and things and much better off in a more creative area. It was a great relief when I finally got a break in a commercial film house as an assistant editor.

What sorts of things were you editing?
I was working at Kingcroft where they made PR documentaries as well as commercials – *Wheat Growing in the Wimmera, Wine Growing in the Barossa Valley* – and I was very lucky because they used to let me cut them and I was allowed to take my time with them. Actually I got that job on totally false pretences. In my desperation to get a job I started writing these letters that got quite over the top – 'save me from the dim-sim bar' or something. I used to write them on brown paper – dim-sim wrapping – and Nick Beauman, the editor who's cut all my films, wrote back and said he didn't have any work but he loved the paper. Nick had mentioned me to Kingcroft because I was this girl who wrote on the brown paper, and the day I started they

said 'oh, you used to work with Nick Beauman?' and I said 'no, not really.' Somehow they thought that he recommended me because I used to be his assistant. I remembered the advice of one of my waitressing colleagues and decided to embellish the truth, so I said 'no, I'm just up from Melbourne, but I used to work with Fred Schepisi.'

As I said, in that year a few things had hit home. One was that there are very few people in this life who do what they really want to do and actually get paid for it. I mean, a lot of people in this film company never talked about film, they weren't interested in cinema or in themes. They'd just be talking about buying their boat or paying off their house or whatever. I came to realise how much a camera cost a day and that you needed a cameraman to make a film – it was all a great shock. I realised that filmmaking was very important to me, that it was something I wanted to keep doing, and I wished I could have had my last year at Swinburne again with my new awareness. So that was why when I saw the ad in the paper for a one-year directors' training course at the newly established Australian Film and Television School, I really wanted to do it.

Film School Number Two: The Australian Film and TV School

So when you went to the Film School, did you have models of the sorts of films you wanted to make?
I remember I'd read about Truffaut and how he'd made notes about real life, so I took around my note book and wrote things like 'fat man in phone box' or whatever. But I started with an open mind really. I knew I wanted to learn and I particularly wanted to learn a lot more about working with actors. The Film School had written to lots of Australian writers – David Ireland, Hal Porter and so on – asking if they had anything like a short story or part of a book that they'd allow us to make into a film. And that's where I found *One Hundred a Day* which was part of an Alan Marshall novel *How Beautiful Are Thy Feet*. That was my first film there.

Were you working with professional actors and technical people?
Yes, that was the great benefit of it for me at the time. I was very lucky
because that course came along at the perfect time in my career – I
still had the naiveté to think I could go out and make films, and I'd had
a year to get a lot of the technical things underway. I used to think 'if
only Nigel could see me now, lacing this projector' – I had always
been very slow at picking up technical things and I used to be held up
as a class joke after the 'how to lace a projector' lesson.

What was it that drew you to One Hundred a Day? *Was it the theme,
the story of the factory girl having an abortion, the setting?*
It was the theme, and also the way it was written was actually very
filmic. The images were coming off the page. You could see it. Those
were the days – the Film School flew me down to meet Alan Marshall.
This story was the first thing of his I'd read and then after I met him I
went away and read the rest of his works. I have great admiration for
him. He was an accountant in a shoe factory in the thirties – and he
had filing cabinets full of notes from that period, snatches of dialogue
and so on. But essentially what I wanted to get across was the strong
human and social concern that is in the story as in all his writing.

*The evocation of the thirties was very well done. Was that
expensive or difficult to do?*
Well, half of the costumes were my dresses! I used to wear a lot of
thirties dresses at the time. And because of the designer training in me
I wanted to have all those things absolutely right. We used to have
make-up students who worked on our crews and I told them I wanted
everything to be absolutely authentic, so they did a research project
and found this mascara that they used to melt on their eyelids like a
wax in the thirties, and some real thirties hair tongs, and so on.

*You use a lot of close-ups and faces that fill the whole frame or
half the frame, which is a style that reappears in many of your
later films as well. Was that a Bergman influence, or . . .*
No, it wasn't an obvious Bergman thing, though from my early
viewing I probably have a huge mixture of Bergman, Truffaut,
Antonioni, and Fellini running around in my head. I think it's my own
interest in faces and the power of faces. It's always been a strong part

in how I cast as well. Still photography had also been a strong interest since Swinburne – I'd spent most of my second year there in the darkroom. I actually feel that *One Hundred a Day* works more as a piece of film than anything else I've ever done.

Really?
Yes. It's in the story itself, because the factory environment is so important. That meant the elements of editing, sound, and photography could carry you and really work your emotions a lot more than in anything else I've done.

The next film was Satdee Night.
That was based around a true event that happened at the house I lived in in Coogee. In fact, one of the girls – the one who keeps getting changed, who can't make up her mind what to wear – is playing me and the car, the old blue Holden, is mine. The actor who plays the main character, lived in the house, and it was his story. At that stage the gay scene was very closed in Sydney and for young gay people their social occasions were very rare – so they were great and very important moments. And just like in the film we all went out to dinner and sent him off to this gay dance saying 'good luck, good luck.' He arrived home the next afternoon and we said 'well, how did you go?' the big Saturday night, and we heard the sad story of how he actually got to the dance and passed out and woke up the next morning on the floor of the Paddington Town Hall covered in streamers and then spent the next two hours trying to get out of the building. I was touched by the story and decided to do that as my documentary.

Were you pleased with the way it turned out?
No, we had a lot of problems with it. It taught me a number of lessons I'm glad I learnt early. The cameraman was one of the few people who really could not cope with a young woman telling him what to do. He couldn't even look at me in the face, plus there were these terrible tensions: I found out later that camera and sound were both Jehovah's Witnesses and they didn't like the subject matter – not only was the character homosexual but part of the story was how he got drunker and drunker. This tension made the actor nervous, and he

started sneaking beer and really did get very drunk. So one lesson was the need to always find a sympathetic crew.

I'd also decided 'alright, I'll improvise scenes and just shoot – it'll give it a real documentary feel.' The main scene is the diningroom scene, and by the time we got to it not only was the lead actor drunk, but everyone else as well. So I had these two crew members who couldn't bear this scene of a room full of drunks, and it just got absolutely out of hand. At one stage I actually had to crawl into the shot and drag the actor out by the leg. I've never let any actors drink again, not even for realism.

How long was it after you left the Film School that you made The Singer and the Dancer?
What happened after I left the Film School was that I got the next lucky break. I had met Tom Cowan at the Film School – he shot *Gretel*, my last film there, and he asked me to be the art director on his film *Promised Woman*. Then *Gretel* was entered in an international student festival at Grenoble in France, and so was *Castor and Pollux*, Phil Noyce's film. The Film School rang and said 'would you like to go to France?' I was overseas for about a year. After the festival Phil and his wife and I travelled round Europe, talking to various student filmmakers we'd met and being tourists. The main thing that I learnt from talking to the other young filmmakers was how lucky we were in Australia to have the government film grant system. So when I got back I wrote a screenplay based on a new story Alan Marshall had sent me called *Old Mrs Bilson* – we had got on very well and kept in contact after *One Hundred a Day* – and put it in for a grant. But I was really broke and needed a job so while I was waiting I worked as art director on John Duigan's *The Trespassers* in Melbourne.

An   Alternative   Film   Scene

Was there an alternative film scene in Sydney along the lines of the Carlton scene that people like John Duigan came from?
While I'd been at Swinburne I had come to Sydney for an Australian independent filmmakers festival at the Sydney Filmmakers Co-op. This for me identified the Sydney filmmakers as experimental – films

by Albie Thoms and Aggie Reid were much more abstract, the 'scratch-blob' films. So when I came up from Melbourne I started going to the Sydney Filmmakers Co-op. There was a real need then for alternative cinemas because there were still very few commercial alternative cinemas. The Co-op films weren't just experimental films, a lot of them were political films that wouldn't be shown anywhere else – this was during the Vietnam period, remember.

How much do you think the tie-up in Australia between exhibition and distribution affects the way things work in the industry?
Well, I think things have changed a lot. At one point it was very hard to get Australian films exhibited at all. Almost impossible, because all the cinemas were owned by the three big chains. David Williams of Greater Union was one of the first to start investing in Australian films and that really caused a breakthrough – naturally the film was shown because the distributor-exhibitors had money in it. And as soon as those films were shown and actually made money, it changed the whole ball game. I should point out, though, that Australian TV is still appallingly behind in any support for independent filmmakers.

MAKING THE MOVIES

The Singer and the Dancer

So The Singer and The Dancer *was a new story by Alan Marshall. That explains why so much of it seems quite modern – the character of the girl who has gone to live in the country with her boyfriend, for instance. She becomes friends with an old woman who has lived through a terrible marriage and is now living with a domineering daughter.*
I should explain what happened. Most of Alan's stories are actually about his own childhood and originally the story was about two boys who used to run into an old woman in the fields in the country. It was essentially a story about how only the very old and the very young can communicate.

I had to rush to get the application in, and when I finally got the money it hit home that it wasn't something that I was passionate about, and I was really in conflict about what to do. John Pleffer who co-wrote the script with me said 'why don't you forget the whole thing about little boys. Make her a young woman. And make it into something you care about.' Not many writers would approve of this, but I wrote to Alan and told him about my difficulties and he said 'fine'. But he said 'I can't write the young couple. You write them and I'll write Mrs Bilson.' So in the film, I'm all the young people and Alan is the old people. I didn't want to do another film set in the past, so rather than do dramatised flashbacks of Mrs Bilson and her husband, I thought 'why don't I have those things happening in the present in the girl's life, so we realise the same things keep happening.' I wanted to play with that idea of the two lives turning the same circles. It's moments like this that you realise the Film Commission have actually been very flexible over the years with their filmmakers: I don't think I told them until after I shot it that it wasn't the screenplay I had given them, and they'd have to look hard to find those two little boys.

Even at that stage I wasn't saying that I wanted to be a feature film director. Though I had worked with Tom Cowan and John Duigan, and a lot of independent features were being made, I hadn't really thought that I'd be making them myself. It was something that was still a bit far away.

How do you feel about the film now?
Well, since *The Singer and The Dancer* I've never written another screenplay, you might have noticed! I saw it recently and felt very embarrassed by it. For me the things that worked were basically in Alan's writing. I felt all the scenes with the kids, all the dialogue I wrote, was very self-conscious, and looking at it in retrospect, God, it seems so heavy handed about relationships. I think the most powerful parts are with Ruth Cracknell, who played the old woman. She was wonderful to work with, and she contributed a lot to the performance.

Did you know people who'd done what the young woman does, retreating to the country, decorating the little farmhouse and so on?

Yes, I knew a lot. Everybody at that stage was carrying on with that sort of bullshit. But I wasn't totally in sympathy with the girl. In my mind the couple were both meant to be poseurs to some extent, and caught up with whatever the youth idea was at the time. But part of the idea was that she would change and get a little bit of humility.

Does she? The film finishes with her going to walk out on the boyfriend who's deceived her, but turning at the gate and walking back to the house.

I was attacked by feminists for making her come back, you know. But I feel the most successful thing about that film was how many people were stirred and angry because they wanted her to walk out. It was funny later on when I tried to sell the film in America to TV people – when they handed the film back they would all say 'why didn't she walk out?' It was the one way I knew people actually watched the film. I was still thinking about it when I shot the scene, but I thought that it was too easy for her to go. She should come back. And it fitted the pattern of going round and round in circles – all my cliché window shots and things.

Your sister worked on The Singer and The Dancer *too. Has she been through the same training as you or did she get involved because you were involved?*

Sue, my sister, went to Swinburne a few years after I did and did graphic art, then she swapped to photography. I asked her to work as my assistant when I worked as art director on *The Trespassers*. Then she started working freelance in art departments. We probably did get too carried away doing up that little hippy house. But it was part of the girl's character that she really did try and wanted to play the game to the fullest extent, to make it the perfect farmhouse. I suppose Sue and I had all that training together, you see, cutting out the silver paper for the costumes for our pantomimes in the garage. So we had this long-established trusted working relationship.

What happened with the distribution of The Singer and The Dancer? *There were difficulties, weren't there?*

Yes. It was probably a very good experience for me because I produced *The Singer and The Dancer* and even though I got the grant it still wasn't enough money to make it. I really had to do all those things of ringing people and trying to get them to work for less money, then I finally had to market it and I think that was a great learning exercise. It was originally taken up by Columbia pictures but it didn't do nearly the business they hoped in Melbourne so they stalled about releasing it in Sydney and finally I took it away from them.

At that stage one of the project officers at the Film Commission was trying to put together some packages: a lot of filmmakers had made fifty-minute dramas with the aid of grants, and he came up with the idea of putting them together in double bills and trying to get some theatrical release. And he suggested that we run with *Love Letter From Teralba Road,* Stephen Wallace's film. I really left it in his hands and went overseas again, in search of this mythical campus circuit in America that might buy the film. The only postal address I had was in Rome, and when I got there about six months later there were all these telexes and letters saying that we'd done record business – we'd broken suburban records and there were queues around the block of the Union Theatre. We had great support from the Australian critics; I think it came just at a time when they wanted something contemporary. And it was a good double: *Teralba Road* is a fine film and I was lucky to be running with it – we were different and yet compatible. So a lot of people went to see it who wouldn't normally have gone to see an independent, low-budget Australian film.

But in fact we never made any money – it turned out the deal with the cinema was a rip-off. Through that experience I realised the problem of that 50-minute length. Unless you can find something for a double bill, an audience needs more in a programme. That was when I realised that I had to make feature films if I wanted to keep making a living out of drama films.

What was it like trying to sell it overseas? It wasn't as easy as you hoped?
I think I imagined people would make their minds up immediately – that was probably my biggest lesson – they'd be stalling and there you are trying to survive on ten dollars a day. And I went off with one print and one cassette and of course they all wanted to hang on to it.

The American television stations had no interest at that stage in Australian drama – they'd all tell me next time I should put in two American actors and I'd have more hope. Finally when I got to London I realised I needed an agent who would keep ringing them and circulating the prints, and after that a number of sales were made to TV stations in Europe.

My Brilliant Career

How did you come to direct My Brilliant Career?
Margaret Fink's first production was *The Removalists* in 1975. I'd done some work in the art department, and she'd asked me to read the book as a friend and say whether it would make a good film. I'd never heard of the author, Miles Franklin, before, and I read it and said 'yes, I think it could, but it would be a big film.' A couple of years and a couple of films later Margaret came back to me and said 'I want you to do it. I want a woman to direct it.' Margaret had never been very impressed with *The Singer and the Dancer* and said 'I want you to make it like *One Hundred a Day.*' I took it on because I liked the book and also because I did think it was important that a woman made it. I thought it could be bungled by a lot of men. Even male friends of mine who read it would say things about Sybylla, the central character, that showed they didn't see her the same way I did. They found her annoying and egotistical, and while I could see all those things, I could see why she was like that.

At the time, though, I thought that I was nowhere near ready to do a big film like that – I really thought that I should do a low-budget feature like John Duigan's or Tom Cowan's, so I was secretly hoping that the script would take a long time to write. In fact it did, because it took Margaret a long time to raise the money, and when it finally came to the crunch I had spent almost two years on and off working on the script with Eleanor Witcombe, and I couldn't let it go. I didn't want anyone else to do it because by then I was just about living it. It was mine.

How clear were your ideas about how the film should look?
Very clear. The overall look was planned extensively with both

Luciana Arrighi and Don McAlpine. But of course things like all those dark skies were pure luck. We shot a lot of the exteriors either in the early morning or the late afternoon. It was something that I learnt way back at Swinburne when I saw a lot of the Swedish films from the early seventies – the reason they all looked so lovely was because everything was done when the light was low, slanting and catching people. Maybe I'm wrong to try to put that European look into my films but I hate the harsh light of the middle of the day and I think it's very hard to photograph people in it sympathetically. But that can be quite a limiting thing for a filmmaker. On scenes like Judy Davis and Sam Neill's first kiss by the river it becomes very hard on everybody, because you only have that light for a short time and it goes very rapidly. It's also very hard to get matching shots for continuity, because late afternoon light drops so rapidly. There are a lot of things I do in my films that are very hard on my actors, and it's a delicate balance between me and my eye and them and the performance.

It must be quite hard to produce those difficult, intimate bits of acting at seven o'clock in the morning.
Yes. Often we all take a bit of time to warm up. Generally as a person I'm a very slow starter but somehow when I'm on a shoot I wake up like a bolt of lightning.

There are other limiting things about Australian schedules and budgets: for instance, in the scene where Judy Davis, who plays Sybylla, dances around in the rain with her hat off. It turned out we couldn't afford the rain machines we'd originally planned to use, so the local fire brigade was called down to assist. The Queanbeyan fire brigade hadn't had much experience in creating rain for film and the first blast from the hose actually knocked Judy straight over, it hit her so hard. It's meant to be like she's reading the book and looks up and there are these delicate drops falling. It was very lucky that I was shooting with two cameras and Don McAlpine, the director of photography, was on the second camera and got a few shots of the water hitting the pond and her hat. That was selected as a clip to be run before the film was shown but for me that was always the most embarrassing sequence – we only had one take and somehow I had to go from all these shots of her sitting reading by the tree to all these shots of her dancing around in the rain. Luckily she kept going after she was knocked over by the water, because her hairpiece, which was waist length, would have taken at least an hour to dry, and as the budget couldn't afford another hairpiece we couldn't rush her quickly into another wardrobe and have another go at four drops falling – that was it. So even with the great planning of these wonderful shots quite often they're not there on the screen – that was one moment that was really saved in the editing room.

But I know I've got to be careful because I think the pictures in my films can become too pretty. I basically want to tell the story, I don't want to detract from that – I don't want people going 'oh, isn't that a lovely landscape!' But at the same time I feel that mood really heightens the drama and that's the balance that I try for. For the interiors I wanted a richness and a feeling of the light coming from the real source – the window or a candle – and a lot of the sequences demonstrate Don's real mastery because we were working with very low light levels, some of them just about candle light, and a little fill. We all worked together on that, and on thinking about the colours and so on that would be right for particular scenes.

Do you ever think about paintings when you're thinking about how you want something to look?
With *Brilliant Career* it was funny because at our first meeting Luci and I both pulled out our postcards of Australian paintings, and we found half the ones we'd each chosen were the same. The strongest influences were from the painters of the time, the 1890s, and there are actual costume details that I could show you, colours and patterns that were from patterns in a Tom Roberts' painting. We weren't just using paintings – we'd done a lot of research into the period.

You did a lot of that research yourself?
Eleanor Witcombe, the writer, had a fantastic library about the period, and I used to go there and read while she was writing the script. When Luci came in, the art department did much more extensive research, but it was important for me because I felt I was totally foreign to that period. As I said, when I was young I actually had a reaction against Australian literature, so it was quite a joke that the first Australian feature film I did was set on a sheep station. I mean, I'm an urban Australian and very proud of it and I'm one of

those people who was always saying, 'why can't we do contemporary stories about where the majority of Australians are?'

I read a lot to find details such as whether an Australian accent had developed by then, and all the social mores and details of behavior. And I also read to understand Miles and Sybylla. I read everything that she talked about, all the writers that she'd loved – they were all the writers I'd refused to read when I was growing up, Banjo Paterson and Henry Lawson, and so on.

At one stage, because there was so much reaction against period films we thought maybe we should update it visually to the 1920s or 1910s but when I started reading I realised that Miles was very much a woman of her time, and the more I read the clearer it became to me that for her that was always the greatest period of her life. It was the period of the first birth of Australian nationalism and she was very much a part of it and very proud of being a part of it. So it seemed almost sacreligious to think about moving it a few years either side. And as well it would denigrate her thoughts as a woman, because there she was out in the bush having had no contact with anything in the outside world like the suffragettes and through the book she was working this thing out all on her own – 'well, I should be equal and why can't I do all those things?' That became very important to me.

Were there any difficulties working on the script?
Well, basically Eleanor and I worked very happily on the script, until the last draft, but finally Margaret and I felt there were some shortcomings in the end product and we had a script editor rework it. Eleanor was upset about it, understandably, and she has never forgiven me. It was a very difficult thing to do. Of course there are still major parts of the script that are Eleanor and her ideas.

There's a difficult balance about putting something that's set in the past onto a modern day screen. Judy, Sam and I reworked the whip scene ourselves the weekend before we shot it; there were things like that that were very delicate because they were very melodramatic and could so easily have gone over the edge and sent the audience into laughter. I still think there are some scenes that are a little stagey and for me the film's greatest failure is when people come to me and say 'why didn't she marry him?' Maybe that's casting, maybe half the audience wanted them to end up together because Sam Neill was so attractive.

How difficult a choice is it for her – does Sybylla ever seriously consider marrying Harry?
Well, it would have been a nice life. He was rich and ...

But did she love him?
No, she didn't and that's what I wanted people to understand – that he wasn't the right one for her. I think she does say something like that in an actual line of dialogue, but I think the audience loved him more than she did.

There are a number of points where she makes him – and us – believe that she is really interested in him. Is she just teasing him?
No, no, she's desperately sexually attracted to him. If Sybylla could have had a good fuck with Harry it would have been a very happy ending. I find it very ironic that I've had medals from the Catholic Church in America and reviews in the Catholic newspapers in America saying it was a sin to miss it! I mean, really I thought that would have been the best thing to happen to them, but of course it couldn't because of the times and that was the tragedy. It could have been a great affair but unfortunately they would have had to get married. Every time she looked at him she knew that she wanted him, that she desired him, but she knew that for a life together he was the wrong person and he'd never really understand her. Also considering the period, she would have had children quite soon and would have found it very hard to be a lady novelist.
   Basically a lot of it was about sexual tension and that was something that we found in the book that I don't think Miles understood about herself. It's a difficult project to translate a book written by a sixteen year old. I mean, the book has some amazing parts that are very truthful, about her family and her life, and other parts that are absolute fantasy. Someone said 'why don't you do it as a send up of a sixteen-year-old's story', but I took *My Brilliant Career* and turned it a little into my story. A lot of people have said to me 'did Miles ever marry? Maybe she was a lesbian.' Maybe that's true, who knows. But I decided my story was to be about a woman who had a lot of potential and really did like men, and did want to be in love, but also

wanted to have a career and fulfill herself and her own creative potential. It's very interesting when you read her descriptions of Harry in the book – there are literally descriptions like 'the material clung tightly over his thighs,' which she probably got from romantic novels of the time. In reality I don't think that there was a Harry.

What sort of relationship did you have with your investors?
I have never met any of the private investors, and we had no major creative interference from the New South Wales Film Corporation or Greater Union who were our major investors – except that Margaret Fink and I had to fight very hard for that ending. David Williams, the General Manager of Greater Union, felt that women audiences wouldn't be able to handle it if Sybylla and Harry didn't end up together. We both said 'look, if you want us to change the story to have them end up happily together, then there's no point in even starting because that's what it's about.' And he said 'well, can't there be a way, can't Harry look back over his shoulder for one last searing look.' And we really did con him a bit, because Margaret was worried that we were going to lose them, so we said 'alright, yes, yes, we'll have Harry looking back.' So what Sybylla says in the final scene with Harry is 'not now' – and of course if you're really romantic you might say ten years later they'll be walking down a street in Paris and they'll see each other across the crowded boulevard.

I had to push that line very heavily at one stage because things did get quite sour – someone told Greater Union that I'd changed the ending and they weren't really going to end up happily ever after. So representatives of the investors came down to the set with this typed-up thing saying 'these were the original words in the last draft and these are the different words and we think you've put this in – and they're going to pull out their money'. So I had to change one line, I put in a line that's an innuendo – where she says 'not now but almost'. That's the sort of pressure that makes directors end up in a nursing home, having that sort of thing arrive at your tea break.

Anyway, at the very first screening we ran for Greater Union and the NSWFC, David Williams, to give him his due, turned around and said 'well, you've been a naughty girl but you're right, it works. You've moved me by telling me she wrote the book.' And that was what I wanted – the final thing was that people would feel triumphant

that she did something. I didn't want them to feel triumphant about
the final kiss in the sunset, it was much more important to have her
alone in the sunset with her package.

*How do you feel about all of Sybylla's pronouncements about
marriage? A lot of them do sound very adolescent.*
They're meant to, she was an adolescent! In our script we stood back
and made her a character who was often still very young and often
quite objectionable. I think we always knew that it was going to be a
hard part to cast – because you had to both love and hate her. She is
an egomaniac and often quite blinded, but she grows up in the film
and matures.

*Was it very hard to find a Sybylla? Casting is obviously some-
thing you care about and take a lot of time with. How did you find
Judy Davis?*
Well, we were casting on and off for almost a year. We didn't see Judy
at all in the first auditions, and I hadn't seen her final year play at
NIDA, when I believe she played Juliet with Mel Gibson playing
Romeo – I'm sorry that I missed the experience. It was very
unfortunate because I'd cast somebody after six months, who had
seemed the best of everyone we'd seen, and she and I had been
swapping books about the period and I went to horse-riding lessons
with her and so on. But when we did the 35mm screen tests, which I
thank the NSWFC for insisting on and paying for, we suddenly
realised that she just wasn't going to work in the part. Margaret Fink
and I looked at each other and knew that she was going to be wrong.
But if I'd been on my own I couldn't have done it, I wouldn't have been
tough enough to smash the hopes of someone who really thought
they had the part for six months. It was a terrible decision and it was
with Margaret's support that we went and spoke to her agent and said
'we're sorry but it didn't work.'

You spoke to her agent rather than to her?
Yes, and that was a terrible mistake – obviously the first thing she did
was to ring me up crying on the phone. So I learnt a lot of things at
that time and one of them is that you can't evade responsibility if you
are going to do something to somebody that's very hurtful. There's

no buffer about it and there's no way you can get anybody else to take
that load. Another was to always base final casting decisions on a
35mm screen test. People are very different on the big screen.

Judy came in a couple of days later and her audition was just
fantastic. She read the speech to Harry at the end about what Sybylla
wanted in life, which at the first read brought tears to my eyes. After
she left the room the casting director and I just hugged each other.

Did you have any trouble finding the man to play Harry?
Yes, we did. It's always been a problem – there are very few young
leading men in Australian theatre and film. I finally saw Sam Neill in
the New Zealand film by Roger Donaldson, *Sleeping Dogs,* at the
Sydney Film Festival and rang Margaret about him, and thank
heavens that worked out. The funny thing is Greater Union wanted
me to see one of the sex symbols of the day, but he turned it down
because he didn't want to play a role where he was rejected by a
woman.

*One of the interesting things in the film is that Sybylla is not a
beautiful woman. She's very striking, but she's not beautiful in
the classic movie sense. And in the film there's quite a lot about
prettiness and the process of making herself pretty. In so many
films the way women look is* assumed *and is never a subject.*
Yes, well that was a strong part of the book. I can still remember the
line she says: 'and then there was an age when I discovered I was a
woman – and not just that but, alas alack, an ugly woman.' That was
my whole subtext in the story, but I've had male friends who've read
the story and say that I copped out by casting Judy because Sybylla
should have been uglier. I said 'you don't understand, she was
probably okay.' There were men all the time who were interested in
her. What she discovered at that time was that she didn't fit into
conventional ideas of beauty – she went through a process that every
woman goes through at puberty of suddenly realising how important
their looks are, and how they're meant to be this or that and 'if only I
didn't have this or that.' The most beautiful women still think they're
ugly or think there's something wrong with their nose or elbow or
their lips. I've just done a documentary for Channel Seven on the
subject, about fashion models, called *Not Just a Pretty Face.* So it's

something that I think is very important and it is something that men don't generally understand.

Two   Doccos

You've made two documentaries about young working-class girls. Can you tell me a bit about them? The first one, Smokes and Lollies, *was made back in 1975.*
It was one of six documentaries that were made by the South Australian Film Corporation with women directors. When the producer rang me up she had already decided that she wanted my film to be about what it was like to be a fourteen-year-old girl. I think they selected me because I've always looked a lot younger than I am and they thought I could go out and mingle with fourteen year olds and not be noticed. At the beginning we all thought that fourteen year olds were going to be a revelation, a new free-living generation.

I went along to a drop-in centre, and ran into these three girls. They were the only girls in this drop-in centre of forty Greek boys. I found out later that they thought that the researcher was my mother and I was coming to join the group, that I was a bit of opposition. In the conversation that evening a few things came out. Firstly they asked how old I was and found out that I was actually over twenty, and the second thing they asked me was 'are you married?' I was surprised and said 'no, why, am I over the hill?' And they went 'yes'. And I said 'why, when should I be married?' And they said 'eighteen'. They were very alive and funny. The researcher and I spent a week with Kerry, Josie and Diana and the girls themselves planned what they wanted to say about being fourteen. But the film ended up a bit of a tragedy. It's not my final cut, and I was very upset – there are things in it that I'm really unhappy about, out-takes have been included and so on.

How did the subsequent film, Fourteen's Good, Eighteen's Better *come to be made?*
Well, the girls had talked so much about being eighteen in the original film that I said to them 'alright I'm going to come back and see.' They'd thought that to be married at eighteen would be the perfect life, because you'd have all the freedom you wanted. *My*

Brilliant Career had just been sold for a record fee, and on the strength of that my agent Hilary Linstead and I approached the TV stations to do the documentary, and Channel Seven agreed to come in with the money. Now I want to follow them up again in a few more years.

How do you feel about the way their lives had gone? Josie had two kids and a broken marriage and Diana was married and about to have a child.

I suppose in a way you could predict a lot of where their lives were going. They did talk quite openly to me when I made *Smokes and Lollies*, so I knew that they were having sexual relations with boys at that time and they knew nothing about contraception (I did have a talk to them about that), so I thought, putting two and two together, it wouldn't be long before somebody was in trouble. The whole film was quite an interesting dilemma. It was the first documentary that I had worked on and it was the first time I realised that there are major ethical decisions involved in making a documentary about real people.

The effect of marriage on individual possibilities seems to be a theme that has concerned you a lot in your work so far.

One thing I do quite consciously have sympathy for is when I feel that people are not realising their full potential and that they are accepting things that they don't necessarily have to accept. But when I read scripts or go out looking for material I don't always start from the theme, sometimes it's just an image or an idea or a character that attracts me. I still feel that I'm very very much a beginner as a filmmaker. And you know I was reluctant to do this interview, because I don't feel that I've done anything that is really even worth discussing. Two feature films is nothing when you look at, say, George Cukor's credits – to think I agonised over the decision about what second film to do: I mean I should worry about it after I've done number 50.

Starstruck

Your decision about a second film was a difficult one?
What happened was that because *My Brilliant Career* had been such
an extraordinary success – and I felt a lot of that was a fluke, I think
success is so much to do with timing – it put a terrible pressure on me
to do the follow-up. I just wanted my first film to be promising, not to
be held up there and revered, and I really do feel that some of the
American reaction to the film was very overblown. Having gone out
and proved I could do it, my biggest worry was 'what if the next one is
a total failure: they'll say "there we knew all along that the
cameraman or the first assistant directed it".' I almost felt that to fail
on the second one was going to be worse than if I'd failed on the first.
And thirdly, I was offered a lot of projects and I realised I was already
categorised very neatly: she makes women's films that are beautiful
and lyrical, with a main female character fighting for identity. I was
sent every possible story that had a main woman character doing
something extraordinary in every part of the world, and always set in
the past. That started to irk me and I thought 'I'll show them, I'll do
something very different.' So I initiated a project that I thought would
be a really heavy political, contemporary film. But as often happens
with original scripts, by the end of the year it had gone through a
number of drafts but hadn't really got much better. And at that stage
Starstruck, which I'd already seen once and been tempted by, came
back under the door.

What decided you to take it?
I heard through some friends of the writer, Stephen MacLean, about
this fantastic script that was unlike any Australian film, a musical
about a precocious fourteen-year-old boy who managed his eighteen-
year-old cousin. And it was originally set in the sixties so I thought it
sounded like fun – obviously it was my era – so I managed to sneak a
copy of the script to read it. I got my agent to ring the producers and
say that I was interested in it and they said 'oh no, we don't want her,
she does those period pictures. She'd be totally wrong for us. It's a
high-energy rock musical.' So it was just a fluke that I ran into
Stephen, who'd been living in England working as a rock journalist,
at a party. I was a bit drunk so I was brave and I shook him and said 'I

wanted that script!' And next day I got a phone call saying that the producer wanted to meet me.

A lot of the dialogue in Starstruck *seems very stylised – it's full of classic thirties musical-type lines like 'life is what you want it to be' and 'you can do anything if you just believe it enough'. Was there a deliberate attempt to be part of that genre?*
Stephen MacLean *was* an Angus. He grew up in a pub in Melbourne where his mother was a barmaid, and rather than dreaming of rock and roll he used to dream of the movies and watch Judy Garland and Mickey Rooney. So yes, that was another level within the script.

What sorts of stylistic issues did that present for you? Obviously it's not naturalistic.
Well, it was difficult. The script could have gone a number of ways. We could have gone in a more extreme direction, doing a total send-up and been much more cynical. But I feel that that genre of film only works in a very limited way, because finally you don't care about anybody. I felt that the kids had to be really believably young and naive, because within Stephen's writing there was always a great love for his people, he wasn't laughing at them.

It was something that I had to be very clear about. On the design side, for example, I had to say 'it's not *Rocky Horror.* 'The first time I went to see a dressing of Aunty Pearl's parlour, it was a sort of kitsch dream. I had it pulled back, saying 'you've got to think of the character, so she's still believable. This shouldn't be like walking into a shop and wondering "will I choose a black lady lamp or three flying ducks?"'

You've said that as a teenager you were a rock and roll fan. Had you had a continuing interest in rock music and the music industry?
Yes, I have been a continuing fan. I was sitting next to a guy on the plane between Los Angeles and New York and somehow we started talking about music and he said 'you know, some people move with the times but I just stay liking the bands that I used to like at eighteen.' Well, I didn't just keep on liking the bands I liked at eighteen. Not that I've got highly sophisticated musical tastes, but

I've always listened to what's been going around and things like the advent of 2JJJ in Sydney have kept my listening up to date. In the late seventies there suddenly seemed to be a lot of interesting music in Australia.

There are two strands to the treatment of the music business in Starstruck. *One is to do with kids' obsession with rock and roll, and the other is to do with the fascination with fame and stardom and celebrity. Were those the things that attracted you as themes?*
The thing that most interested me in the script was the relationship between Jackie and Angus and their family. For a long while I was in two minds about whether Jackie should even be a success at the end, but I felt that the whole sense of the film was the optimism and a real love of people so it was important that there was a happy ending – though I think now it was maybe a trifle bland.

Finally I think that the film in a very simplistic sense was in praise of free spirits. There are a lot of rock movies about the fame and the pill-popping and the selling-out for the record contract but that really wasn't the purpose of *Starstruck*. I would have liked just a slightly more bitter twist. I thought you should feel that once Jackie had got fame, that she had grown up and left Angus: their closeness and their relationship had finally got her where they both wanted her to go, but that meant that their relationship was over. I'm sure that comes out, but I would have liked it to be a little bit tougher.

How was the decision made to use the Swingers as the band and to get Phil Judd to do the music?
One of my greatest regrets about the entire film was that the music was got together in a very chaotic way. There had to be a band that was Angus' favourite band and I pushed very strongly to find a band that fitted in with Angus' personality: it shouldn't be a band that was built around a sexy male lead, they had to be a bit bent. I very strongly pushed for Split Enz, but that turned out to be impossible. But I certainly don't want to denigrate Phil Judd's talent because his getting involved was very fortunate for us and I think his input to the film was wonderful.

In our search for song writers, the original music director and I found that very few people had the ability to write songs around a story, a drama, and a required emotion. We'd specify 'this song should affect people in a pub and get them happy and make them dance', and songs would come in that were like something that you'd play at a funeral. So things were getting very desperate: I soon learned that good songs are a rare commodity.

The Swingers single *Counting the Beat* had just come out, and I thought that they would fit the bill, being a little different and a little eccentric. The first time I met Phil Judd he stared at the wall and didn't speak to me. Their manager said 'oh, but they're wildly enthusiastic.' But at the second meeting Phil did actually speak, and even asked a few pertinent questions about the lead-in in the dialogue. By that stage I'd heard so many theme songs, I was saying 'maybe we shouldn't have a theme song, maybe nobody can write a theme song that doesn't sound corny, maybe it's impossible.' So I was amazed when Phil's *Starstruck* theme actually arrived, and I was thrilled with it because I think he managed it in a way that wasn't too cute.

For me *Starstruck* would have been a better film if we hadn't had a drama with our first musical director dropping out halfway through. The official statement was that it was a disagreement in musical tastes with me, and he didn't have the sort of patience to work with someone inexperienced like Jo Kennedy, who plays the lead, Jackie. By that stage all the production machinery was rolling, and rehearsals were scheduled with the choreographer, who was only available for a short time.

Total chaos was threatening, so I was thrilled when Phil wrote *Starstruck*, and they offered to do some more. I sent them off to write the water-ballet music. I said 'I know it's too much to ask, but if you really want to know when we need it, it's tomorrow.' And sure enough they turned up at one o'clock in a taxi with the tape and it was *Tough*. We listened to it once, the choreographer grabbed the tape, and raced down the stairs to the rehearsal. It isn't the way to make a musical, though I have heard since of similar things going on in even greater projects than our little production. I never want to work that way again. I don't feel it was fair to the songwriters, the choreographer, or to the performers, but it was really desperation in the end.

The look of Starstruck *is very consistent and coherent as a style. How did you approach that aspect of the film?*

I was very worried about how the kids were going to look, knowing how quickly youth styles change and how long it takes to get a film out. It was something I talked about at length with both the designers. I chose Brian Thomson, who was the designer for *The Rocky Horror Show,* to do the sets, I wanted slightly heightened reality, and Brian was a great mind for ideas, so his designs say a lot more than just being pretty colours. Luciana Arrighi had done all the original design for *Brilliant Career* and she wanted to do the clothes for the same reasons as me, I think: to prove that she wasn't just lace and soft candlelight. It was impossible to guess what was going to be in fashion in eighteen months, so we decided to design our own things around the two characters – ideas about Angus playing the manager, for instance, with the Hollywood manager's gilt jackets. With Jackie we really went to town, putting together as many offbeat things as we thought the character would've done but always trying to retain the feeling of something she'd cooked up at home.

How did you approach the cinematography? You were working with Russell Boyd again, as on The Singer and the Dancer.

We wanted a sort of hard edge and brightness in the look. There's a theory that comedy should be brighter on the screen, so you don't do the sort of moody *Brilliant Career* thing. But I didn't want to go for the total fifties look, where it is absolutely overlit, because we needed some feel of the story being set in a real place. So that was the basic idea, with things like the rooftop pool scene being shot in the evening – the Sydney skyline at dusk when all the lights are on is just a fantastic time.

Did you work closely with David Atkins on the choreography of the musical numbers?

Yes, I would watch rehearsals and try and explain what I wanted in my limited vocabulary. What I'd always wanted was for the dance to be original, for it to have a sense of humour and a lot of energy, and I didn't want it to be pretty. Not many choreographers would allow a director to come in and comment on this and that step but we got along very well. He'd go off to put it together and I would go in later with Russell Boyd and the camera operator and look at the rehearsals and talk about the ways to shoot it. No one had ever worked on a musical before, and everybody on the crew was really excited by it. It's amazing the feeling that's created on a set by having music going all day: it got everybody going and even though it was hard work, people really enjoyed working on the dance numbers.

Were you influenced at all by the rock-clip phenomenon, which has really exploded in the last couple of years?
I wanted to react against it. One of the producers suggested using a place in America where you can do a lot of tricksy effects on film, but I felt the thing we had going for us was that it was a real story, with real people, and so we should have real dance numbers, with people really dancing. We tried to capture the feeling that the dance was happening within the actual span of time, and to avoid going into total fantasy.

How was it working with the young actors Ross O'Donovan and Jo Kennedy who'd never acted before?
What I was most worried about is that the filmmaking process is so drawn out and can be very boring. There are long waits and then suddenly you have to come up with instant energy and be the part. And I had them coming to me halfway through saying 'nobody told us how boring it would be' and how awful it was to get up at 6.30 every morning. So there were extra conflicts that made it harder for them to be the bright, zestful, energetic young things they were before it all started.

I had to watch Jo go ahead and make major errors and mistakes, a lot of which I felt were damaging to the film – it was very hard sometimes for me to keep my patience. We'd say 'you know it will show on your face the next day if you party all night,' but it wouldn't make any difference. Doing *Starstruck* was the first time I actually felt old. All these years that I've been doing these youth culture films and everyone had said 'oh, she should do the one about the fourteen-year-olds because she's a teenager who won't grow up. I had thought I should do a youth film before I got too old, while I still understood a bit about what's happening with rock and roll. But going out with an eighteen and a twenty-one-year-old, for the first time in my life I felt 'yes, I have grown up'. In the end I was walking around saying all these platitudes like 'you can't tell them anything, they have to learn it themselves.'

It's quite a responsibility, taking inexperienced young people out of their ordinary lives and into that kind of celebrity.
That's true. Even apart from adapting to the work process there are the problems of moving two people away from their home and their friends for quite a long time. I knew that the film was going to have an effect on them personally. Suddenly they were up there on the screen and they attracted many more fans than Judy and Sam had in *My Brilliant Career* because they were reaching a younger fan audience. Poor Jo would be on the bus going to the dole office and people would ask for her autograph. It's very difficult to be getting that adulation while the reality for actors in the Australian film industry is that good parts are very rare in most age ranges, let alone for teenagers. The producers have been extraordinarily responsible to both Ross and Jo and their families: their and my involvement has gone on much longer than it normally would. My advice to most young actors is 'forget it' – go back to school and if a good part comes along maybe do it. But both of them were bitten by the bug: once you've had a taste of that sort of work, you want more.

REFLECTING ON DIRECTING

Constructing the Pictures

The composition of images seems to be an important part of filmmaking for you. Do you imagine every shot before you go onto the set?
Generally I do. I always try to find images that are important to me that I then work into the whole frame of the story. Obviously there are always certain dialogue scenes where it's better to really let the actors have a free range. I storyboard all my films – every shot. They don't always come off – often the camera operator or the director of photography

have a better idea at the time, but for me it's really important to know beforehand what I'm aiming for. I do little drawings – the actors are generally very amused by them, especially when they notice I have expressions on their faces. I say 'yes that's right, you just smile like that.' Little stick figures with smiles and frowns and things. Obviously this became quite taxing moving from small films into larger films, finding the time to do them all. I plan the whole cutting of the thing as well – it's actually story boarded almost like a finished film in my head – but of course many things are changed and improved during editing.

Not One of the Boys

You've talked a lot in the course of this interview about the contribution that different people make in the production of a film, but you are also identified with a position that emphasizes the director as the most important person in the filmmaking process.
I've argued the importance of the director in the context of definitions of Australian content and what makes a film Australian, which has been an issue in relation to which films should get tax concessions. It's quite obvious from my background, my feeling and the sort of films that I try and make that I believe that the director really does control the major creative decisions in the film. So in the content debate if you ask what makes a film Australian, I can never question that if the director and the writer are not Australian then how can that vision on the screen possibly be Australian.

One of the things that has emerged from both the sixties political movement and the women's movement has been an interest in more collective styles of organisation and work. Do you think that sort of approach can be used in the area of film?
Honestly I don't think it can, because finally somebody has to make up their mind and say yes or no. Filmmaking is a myriad of decisions from beginning to end over the tiniest details. Now I can see on very rare occasions that perhaps two people who were very close and had a similar vision could do it. But I have actually seen collaborative projects that have come to very grim and bitter ends – and a couple of them were women's projects – because finally the strongest member of the group took over.

I remember one Australian film that was made with a lot of support from women's groups, and during the actual filming they would have a meeting to discuss every shot. A friend of mine – a man – was shooting it and he wasn't allowed to be in on these discussions in one scene they were all meant to be running towards him but they'd just had a meeting where they'd decided they were going to run the other way, so he was pointing the camera and they all just sort of ran past him and out of the shot in two seconds. It was just chaos.

But I like to say that my films are nothing without my editor, my directors of photography, first assistant, designers, and the writers and producers. I don't like working alone. I really need feedback from people and I am often helped greatly when I've gone off the rails. I've never made a film where I didn't get a contribution from every member of my crew, but finally somebody has to filter that information and keep balance by saying yes, no. Because for me the best films are those where I feel one person is telling me something in a balanced way.

The role of the director is very much a leadership position in relation to the set and the crew. How would you describe your style in that role?
I haven't got one. I mean occasionally people have tripped over me and realised that I was the one who was whispering the commands to somebody. It was something that only came to me step by step, and it really didn't hit me until I made *My Brilliant Career,* where I went from a crew of about fifteen on *The Singer and The Dancer* to a crew of 54. And actually I'm quite inhibited amongst a lot of people and I was absolutely terrified at the start. I remember when the Australian press came down to the set of *My Brilliant Career,* all writing stories about this freak woman director. A lot of them still had that idea of the old days of somebody with jodhpurs and a megaphone, and they were so disappointed because in fact it's the first assistant director who shouts all the commands. But among the men I know as directors there are a lot of even shyer, more inhibited people than me going out there and stuttering their wishes in somebody's ear.

I suppose what finally got me through that film, and made me stop worrying about whether anyone was paying me any attention, was realising that everyone is standing around waiting to be told what to do and *somebody* has to tell them. I probably learnt that when I was a student and I used to take wedding photographs on the weekend to pay my way through Swinburne. I remember the first time I went out I was absolutely terrified – but when they all came out of the church and were standing there I realised that they were actually more terrified than me. Because they didn't know what to do. So that was the first time I actually had to get up and direct and say 'where's the mother and the new mother-in-law, in here, move in, over there.' I realised that being a leader isn't something you need to be afraid about, it's often just that people are delighted to get some guidance. And if you can have that together in your head then you can get through the day.

Were there difficulties for you as a woman working with the crew and having them accept your authority and respect your judgements.
I'd learnt my lessons over the years of making short films and I have this mental list of types of people to avoid. There are a lot of men over the age of about 45 who have such inbred chauvinism they will never be able to take one word of command from me, or even have proper discussions about what's possible. I've also come into conflict with women who have worked for a long time in a male-dominated industry as supporters of the great male talent. Some of them find it impossible to work with a woman director, because they believe that they're there to support the wishes and whims of this great male god. For me personally that's even harder to cope with than the men. But in fact I've had fantastic support from some men who are over 45 – I should name them, but they're possibly hiding their ages. I can understand people being envious of me, being a lot younger and having the power and the job that they may have wanted and sought after for years, so I've been really lucky that a lot of the men and women that I've worked with have been fantastic people to collaborate with.

A Woman in the Australian Film Industry

The film industry in some ways seems a very gossipy, competitive industry. Do you think women cope in that system differently from men?
I think that the gossiping and back-stabbing may come from the fact that it's a freelance industry – nobody knows about their next job, so there are great insecurities. Obviously because we're all competing for limited funds, and of all the projects that are running around only a small percentage are made, there are lots of jealousies about who's finally getting the money and for what reasons.

The gossip about *Brilliant Career* was incredible. It was then the biggest film for any first-time filmmaker, and for that filmmaker to actually dare to be a girl and to have a woman producer was just too much for some people. I heard stories back that it was a lesbian film, that for women to be working together they had to be on together. I'm sure Bruce Beresford wouldn't like us to say that about his productions because he generally works with men. Still, I don't think gossip is just an Australian industry affliction.

Do you think being a woman in that environment makes it harder to take?
Well, there are extra pressures on me. Especially during the first film I felt I was being watched by every single member of the industry, and that most of them really did want me to fail. I know that sounds dreadfully paranoid but there was a lot of gossip, firstly that it was outrageous that we were going out with all this money; secondly that it was another boring period film; and thirdly that it was a woman's film with two women working together so it must be going to be against men. I do know people came into the editing room while Nick Beauman was cutting the film saying 'does it cut together?' They thought 'it's made by that young woman, surely it must be a mess.'

I felt that I wasn't just being judged as a young filmmaker going out to make their first film, I was being judged as a woman making a film. If it had failed it wouldn't have been just that I couldn't do it and didn't have the talent, it would have been that *women* couldn't do it, that *women* couldn't stand up to the rigours of the shoot physically, or that *women* couldn't hold a production that large together.

So the people who did back me and never questioned me like Michael Thornhill in the NSW Film Corporation and David Williams at Greater Union and Don McAlpine and Margaret Fink certainly have to be commended for their conviction because there was a lot of backchat around.

You've never been actually involved in the organised women's movement. Have you felt under moral pressure from the women's movement at all?

I was invited along to a few meetings in the early stages of the Sydney Women's Film Group, but at that stage I'd never really been involved in any group activity and disliked meetings, so I didn't go. But the fact that I wasn't there was interpreted as that I wasn't a supporter. By then I'd reached a different stage with my own films so I didn't need them, though I really see the importance for women of mastering all the technical things in an unselfconscious way.

My films were shown as part of women's group screenings, and some of the more radical members criticised my films quite heavily. They said things like my films look too slick and like a man's, or that I had two women characters who didn't love each other. It used to make me very angry because my premise is to try and make something that works as a whole, and I certainly don't feel that the way to take a message to your audience is through a blatant commercial, which is what they're asking me to do. I've always described *Brilliant Career* as soft feminism but it probably has taken its message to a much wider audience than most of the small independent women's films.

But there's always been criticism that implies that because I'm a woman filmmaker I should be fulfilling certain criteria. I find it very annoying and just as sexist to say that as a woman I should only be making films about women and about women's themes, and that they should portray women as always showing the positive sides of sisterhood. That makes me very angry as an artist and a woman, because I feel that I have the right to make films about any subject I like, just as men have. But at the same time, obviously, I do feel a real moral obligation to the women's movement, of which I am a total supporter, which means I would always worry about doing anything in my films that put down women in a sexist way, and I am conscious of that when I'm both writing and shooting my films.

You've said you don't want to be identified as a woman's director, but the films that you've made have almost all been stories about women.
Well, you see that's me as a person. I spent a whole year on a script about seven young boys, and at the end of that time I picked up a script on a young girl and went off and made *Starstruck*. But that's what I'm trying to say – I'm an individual and the things that come out in my films are lots of parts of me and one of the major parts of me is that I'm a woman. But I don't like to be put in a category, I want to feel that all my options are open and that in the next (hopefully) 30 years or so of filmmaking, there will be lots of subjects that I'll cover.

Ranging from the documentaries about the teenage girls to The Singer and The Dancer *to* Brilliant Career *there is a continuing interest in the effect of relationships and marriage on women's lives. How do you feel about those tensions yourself?*
Well, obviously it was a theme that was very important to me, but since I made *The Singer and The Dancer* eight years ago there have been so many films along those lines that it seems really clichéd. I grew up in a very conservative time in the fifties, and despite changes in the sixties most of my school friends got married in their early twenties. When I was growing up it was still the situation that if you weren't married, you were a failure.

Now, I really do think love and relationships are among the most important things in life, but it's tragic when you see people pressured into something that they feel they can never get out of. A lot of my contemporaries married because they were guilty about sex, because they felt 'I've finally done it, I'd better make it legal'. I really don't think that's a great criteria for deciding who you should spend your life with. I really think that it's impossible to say that love will last forever, and I believe that relationships should be a lot more flexible. So that's been my one small rebellion in life, and my mother very disappointedly says that she never saw a daughter down the aisle.

In My Brilliant Career *you present the possibility of having both a
satisfying career and a good relationship as a conflict.*

There were a few things that I wanted to come through in *My
Brilliant Career* that weren't in the book. I made a conscious decision
to give it a positive ending, because that's how I felt reading it – here it
is, she's only sixteen and she's done it, I'm holding the book she wrote
in my hand. That ending was something we added. Another thing was
coming to terms with the question of how plain or pretty, in the
traditional sense, Sybylla was. It's something *I've* come up against
time and time again. When I meet people they look surprised and say
'oh, *you're* the woman director. You don't look anything like I
expected you to look'. I say 'what did you expect me to look like, a
55-year-old hairy monster?' And they really do. The whole thought is
that the only women who do have the sort of careers that take time
and energy are the ones who have missed out on a few of the attributes
to catch a man, so they sublimate all their sexual energy and their
capabilities for love. That was my own statement in *My Brilliant
Career.*

You don't think it's an either/or choice?

I think it's very hard for women. I do think filmmaking's a very tough
and selfish career. It is very hard for me to be a woman director and
maintain relationships. People have often asked me, have you wanted
to be a man? And I never have, it's never entered my head – I never
wanted to kick around footballs and all that stuff anyhow. But the one
area where I think it would be wonderful would be to have a wife in the
traditional sense! How I envy the male directors the way they can go
up to their studies and there's somebody down below looking after
the children or cooking their meals and kissing them goodbye the day
they go off to the shoot.

It is very tough, because unfortunately to be a good director – and
it's something I'm trying to work at – takes all of yourself. It takes all
your mind, all your control, all your energy and there's a period,
generally from early pre-production of a film to the end of shooting,
where you just have to cut off totally. So I think in that way it's easier
to be a male director than a woman, definitely. Personally I've been
very lucky in that I have had rare support from my other half that not
many women in this business get.

I mean, I really did think that if Sybylla had married Harry in *Brilliant Career,* as a Victorian wife she would have had children very early and it would have been impossible. And I do believe that why we have so few real women artists at all levels in history is because women bear the children and finally they bear the conscience about having those children. As much as men can say 'oh but they could have had nurses and this and that' I think that a lot of women's major creative energies have gone into bringing up children. I personally believe that it is a huge commitment to bring a life onto the earth, and that that's probably one of the reasons why in a business as taxing as the film business there are so few women directors.

Is having children something you think about?
I think the best way to put it is I don't think that all people have to have children. It actually annoys me that magazines like *Woman's Weekly* are continually writing triumphant stories about these poor women who have gone to the absolute ends of the earth to find some sort of sperm from a whale or whatever to help them become fertile. I certainly would never want any woman to feel that her life isn't full because she hasn't had children. But I don't know what I'll finally do. I think I'd make a dreadful mother which is one of the things I'm most worried about – I need a first assistant in the home.

The First Feature: Traps for the Unwary

Were there any major surprises or lessons that you learned on My Brilliant Career *as your first feature?*
Luckily I had a very experienced crew and through the help of the cameraman and first assistant I picked up lots of little tricks about trying to get the most out of the day. But at times I was swamped by the technical things, and there were times when my actors needed me more. One of the big things I learned was when to say 'thank you' to people. You know, you feel you're carrying this burden on your shoulders. I'd do a scene in one room and I'd just be walking out into the next one with a despairing look on my face and I'd be pulled up and told 'look, your crew have worked very hard for you in that setup

and you didn't thank anybody,' and I'd just sort of go 'oh! I thought they understood – I *was* happy.' So on a really basic human level I learned a lot about working with a large group of people.

And on an overall level you always learn the most from what's on the cutting room floor. There were a lot of scenes of Sybylla being a governess that were cut out of the film and I learned on a story level that there are some very delicate balances. If somebody's having a bad time, you only need to show that once.

Another weakness is that in a stylistic way the whole section with the McSwat family is totally out of keeping with the rest of the film and that it went a little bit over the top. I know *why* that all got slightly out of control – we were there bogged in this swamp with eight crying children who had never had mud on their feet; my designer was trying to fire the art director and had just thrown a pot of tea over his head at breakfast. There are days like that when you have to try and remember what you are doing and not to be affected by it.

In a positive way, one of the things that I know worked very well was the relationship I had with Margaret Fink. She was a creative producer who was able to come in at the end and tell me things that weren't working. And secondly, I'm really delighted with all the cast in *Brilliant Career,* without exception. That told me once again how important casting is. There's one rule that says it's 90 per cent of your film – well, I don't think it's 90 per cent but it's certainly 60 per cent.

So I learned all those things and I also learned that finally you have to be ruthless and trust your instincts because unfortunately when your film is up on the screen around the world nobody knows about how the rain machine didn't turn up or whatever – ultimately all the audience sees is what you've put on the screen. That is probably the largest lesson I've learned.

Success and the Press

How affected are you by the press?
Well I've certainly been aware of the Australian press and film critics and how it sometimes gets out of hand and affects the people being written about. I realised the effect of the critics even before I made *My Brilliant Career:* Margaret Fink, the producer, had a lot of trouble

raising the money because of a critical trend towards Another Boring Period Picture reviews. Even the Film Commission was infected with it. We were jumping up and down saying 'I'm sorry, it *is* set in the past, but they don't have to be boring.' There are good and bad films in every genre. So I was very frightened that my review heading was going to be Another Brilliantly Boring Period Picture and I used to make jokes about the title and its unfortunate possibilities.

What I try and do, is to know what I want out of a film and to accept the good and bad things in it. But still, sure, we all want good press, for emotional and personal reasons, and also because it encourages an audience to see the movie. I've always thought *My Brilliant Career* was overpraised in a lot of places. I think if you're going to believe the good press, then one day you've got to believe the bad press! So it's better to hang on to a more balanced viewpoint. And you've got to have a few people that you know and trust, because there is a point where you are too close to it. As time passes though, you can pull away and look at it and see all the flaws.

AN AUSTRALIAN OR MID-PACIFIC CINEMA?

You've said that you're more interested in making films about Australia than anywhere else. What is it about Australia that interests you to put into films?
It's not necessarily a strict rule that I will only make films about Australia, it's a much more personal thing. I've read hundreds of American scripts and had lots of offers, and a lot of them are by very good writers. But for me the best films do have an intimacy with people and human behaviour, and both the director and the writer have to know their subject very intimately. And so far I haven't read anything that I've related to in the same way as I relate to Australian material. The Americans find our films refreshing and optimistic and many of them *are* like that. But one of the main things about Australians is their sardonic humour and cynicism – it's strange really, that we have this image in the world as starry eyed and naive.

Sex,   Style,   and   Rock   and   Roll

We've talked about My Brilliant Career, *but how do you feel about the treatment of sexuality generally in Australian films?*
Has it ever been treated? I think it would be a great challenge as a filmmaker to do something that was really erotic and passionate. I'm just trying to think have I ever seen . . . apart from the hideous and coarse treatment in films like *Petersen*. I think the shot in that of Wendy Hughes' bikini pants being pulled down and a hand rising in the frame must be one of the most memorable shots in Australian cinema. *Monkey Grip*, I suppose, is the first to really deal with it, and very bravely I think.

There was a lot of criticism at the one stage of the first batch of Australian films saying that there was no emotion in them, and asking what's wrong with us, why can't we deal with emotions, is it because Australians are inhibited as a people? I think certainly with some of the male filmmakers that is part of the answer; they *are* frightened of emotion and frightened of women, and they hold back. I also think there was a conscious reaction in the seventies to previous melodramatic styles. It was an age of cynicism in cinema and a lot of Australians tried to do that by holding back and never going to the full extent. But to me some of those films are like coitus interruptus: the major dramatic scenes are always happening off the screen and the next thing you find out something happened but they didn't play them, you get the information indirectly, or in captions at the end. I think sometimes that fear of drama is a fear of emotion.

Rock music seems to have been an important influence for you and is central in Starstruck. *Do you think there is a distinctive sensibility that runs through Australian rock music as well as Australian films?*
It's hard to define. Australian bands in the late seventies had a musical style that had more melody and more humour than most of the music that followed the punk period. They seemed to have picked the eyes of all the styles of music that were around and mingled them all. So there's a sixties pop feel and there's a little bit of reggae, and they've put them together in their own way. That slightly tongue-in-cheek

quality has been around for a long time, with bands like Daddy Cool, who were really ahead of their time, and Skyhooks, in the early seventies. It's almost a send-up of the genre, but taking it further and not just mimicking it. There's something very Australian in that sort of humour. I've been asked about the music in *Starstruck* a lot in America. They want to hear about an 'Australian Sound', since Men At Work have been such a success there – they have that melody and cheekiness too.

There is an interesting trend in Australian clothing and interior design towards Australiana, which as a fashion style also has something of that tongue-in-cheek character. Starstruck *certainly seemed to pick up on that.*

Yes, it does have that quality. That's grown a lot since we made *Starstruck*. Then, it was much more an 'in' fringe thing, a sudden interest in Australian icons and images of Sydney, of the bridge and so on. We thought we were very clever. We even thought about using a harbour bridge design as our logo, but I'm glad we didn't because it's become hackneyed – that kitsch postcard send-up look has become quite a popular thing in Australia, at all levels of design.

A lot of it has stemmed from the fashion designers Linda Jackson and Jenny Kee of Flamingo Park, who were the first to use Australian motifs on their clothes, such as koalas on the back of cardigans. And that's being mimicked all over. There really is a distinctive Australian look. I think it's great but at the moment I feel like if I see another Sydney T-shirt, I'll scream.

It's interesting the way *Starstruck* has been accepted overseas. I really thought that nobody would understand that it was tongue-in-cheek. It's a bit of a fluke that an interest in Australia is beginning to catch on: I've been really surprised, because they do get the joke.

Sydney vs Hollywood

Have you been tempted by the notion of working in Hollywood?

I think probably for any director there's a time when it becomes very hard to continually work under the tight disciplines we have here which quite often do add up to artistic compromise. I mean small things like not being able to go away and reshoot a scene that you're unhappy with, or having to roll the cameras when the light's not right because it must be done. And I can certainly understand why directors like Fred Schepisi and Bruce Beresford, having worked here for much longer than I have, have felt the need to go and to grow. Also there is the whole ethos of Hollywood – it is the centre of the English-speaking film industry. And finally of course, the money is so much better, both for film budgets and personally. It's very tempting the way Americans are able to buy up talent; they buy you security and time to work on ideas.

But on the other hand, I've spent time in Los Angeles and spoken to a lot of people about the bad sides, because often with greater money can come greater artistic restrictions and interference. There are very few directors in the world who have the final cut of their films. But for me, any film is two years out of my life and if I'm going to make that commitment and spend that time on something, I don't want it taken away from me and changed for arbitrary reasons.

Are there dangers of those trends happening in Australia?

Well, what seems to be happening here, rather than the films being taken away and being changed at the end, is that the good films seem to be no longer being made. Which is probably even more worrying, because we can all battle and fight compromising situations when you've actually got it in the can. There seems to have been a change in the pattern of films that are being made now as compared to two years ago. At the moment it seems there are fewer *Breaker Morants* and *Devil's Playgrounds* being made. Now that we have government tax concessions for investment in the film industry, our industry too is moving into the hands of the money men. And unfortunately this can ruin the whole creative impulse of a film and it will show on the screen.

A lot of the projects with good directors and producers, people who've produced really worthwhile work before, are simply not being made. It's the films of a much lighter nature, situation comedies or action dramas, that are getting the funding. It's that fifties commercial thinking that says audiences want action, sex, violence and horror. But that thinking is quite out of date – I mean, the films that you see making money all round the world are your *Ghandis*, *E.T.s*, and *Tootsies*. That thinking is coming from people who have very little knowledge and experience of film, and who are basically interested in making money, not in making films. And unfortunately, I think they are the people who are guiding Australian investors into Australian films and I think that could be very very damaging.

The Directors' Association

You've focussed your concern about some of these things into the Directors' Association. How did it start?
Well, the Directors' Association was formed by a key group of Phil Noyce and James Ricketson, who were both at the Film School with me, and Steve Wallace and Albie Thoms. Compared to the first wave of the new Australian directors, who came from very different walks of life, the second group that I'm part of have always been more collaborative. Through the Sydney Filmmakers Co-op a lot of the people had been through a group process before, discussing and analysing films and we've shared resources and tried to help each other along the way.

The producers in this country had formed a very strong association and traditionally had been very good at politicking and at one stage they started bringing in a number of overseas directors. We thought that was very detrimental to young filmmakers, that they'd never get the break that I got or Phil Noyce got at 27 or 28. So out of that and feeling that we all still had a lot to learn about filmmaking, we decided to set up the Association. I've always been in the early key group and I can't quite work out how it happened but I'm the president at the moment. But I'm not going to have enough time to carry on with it now.

A   Man's   World

Is it possible to make generalised remarks about the position of women in the Australian film industry?
Well, at the moment we have, percentage wise, a lot more women producers than most other countries. I think one of the reasons that I got my break, and why there are so many women producers, is that the rebirth of the film industry happened at the same time as the birth of feminism and a new consciousness of the need for independence for women.

In a certain sense anyone with enough nouse can become a producer. Whether you can actually last is another story, because you do have to have very special talents, but basically if you can get the money together and buy a property that's right and get a good director interested, then you're on your way. So a number of women have come in at the top in that way. But it's quite puzzling why there are so few women in drama directing, not only in Australia but in the world, even in America where they have hundreds of film schools. Perhaps because film is such a technical medium women shy away from it because they're frightened they'll never understand all the lights and leads and lenses and so on.

Many of the women working in film in Sydney stem from the Sydney Women's Film Group, which was established in the very early seventies, almost as a branch of the political women's movement. They were women who were very concerned about women's role in society and they wanted to communicate that through film or video. For a time it was a very powerful group, and lobbied for things like the Women's Film Fund so that there'd actually be government money for women writers and producers on films that were exclusively about women's themes. And they pressured the Film School to encourage women to train in all technical areas. So I think they've been a really positive force in the industry. Before, as much as people would say they weren't discriminating against women, they certainly never took them on in apprenticeships and trained them in sound or camera. Some of the younger cameramen have been very helpful though, like Russell Boyd who trained Jan Kenny, the first woman feature film camera operator.

There seem to be a lot of women producers in Australia, but in America that isn't the case at all – why do you think that is?
Well, when I talked to women in a film group in Los Angeles, they applauded me for *My Brilliant Career* saying 'what you've done for all of us is made a film that looks expensive, that looks big.' Even if in the American context the budget wasn't large it certainly was in the Australian context. They told me that's not happening in America – the women directors who've had a break have made low-budget independent films. Even when they get their studio film it's very rarely of a reasonable size or budget.

It is a really insidious sort of discrimination: that men don't really trust women with money. And it's probably something that people couldn't even talk about, they wouldn't say 'oh, well we couldn't let that young thing go out for ten weeks with ten million dollars riding on her back because she might faint in the heat as the camels were approaching.' The Hollywood system works very differently from the Australian system where the money is usually raised in very small lots. In America the money usually comes in one huge lot; it's one studio and one person's – generally one man's – decision. I really think that is one of the major reasons why there are so few women directing feature films.

But also I do believe that this is still a man's world and that any women who has succeeded in any way in the film industry has had to be better than the men. You can be a mediocre male director and still keep making films for the next twenty years but if you're a mediocre woman director you'll never get anywhere. The right to fail is accepted more among men. American directors like Claudia Weil and Joan Micklin Silver made successful independent films but their first Hollywood films were not commercial hits, so they are considered failures. But with a man's second film people would have said 'well, yes, he's definitely got promise but he should've had a stronger scriptwriter' or whatever, and he'd be given his next break.

So how likely is it that you will work in Hollywood in the near future?
Well I have an arrangement with the Ladd Company to offer them first option on anything I want to do. I decided to go with them

because they are a small company and they were the only ones who were willing to invest in something I might do in Australia: all the others wanted me to either produce a film there or to find a script that would be a vehicle for two or three American stars that might be set in Australia. But things have tightened up in Hollywood just as they have in Australia, and the last time I was there the feeling seemed to have changed from 'whatever you want to do' to 'have you got an optimistic, bright, upbeat story?'

Working in Hollywood for itself isn't a major objective though, and even though there are some wonderful actors and writers there, as I said earlier I haven't found anything I want to do so far. If the problems in Australia get worse, and it becomes impossible to raise money for the sort of films I want to make here, then I will go. There have been a few projects that have looked possible, but there's been nothing I've felt passionate about, and I know there's no point in me just taking something on as a job in a half-hearted way. You just wouldn't survive all the trials and tribulations – the actors and the wardrobe lady in tears, the sun going down, and the wind machine not working before you've finished the shot – without that passion guiding you.

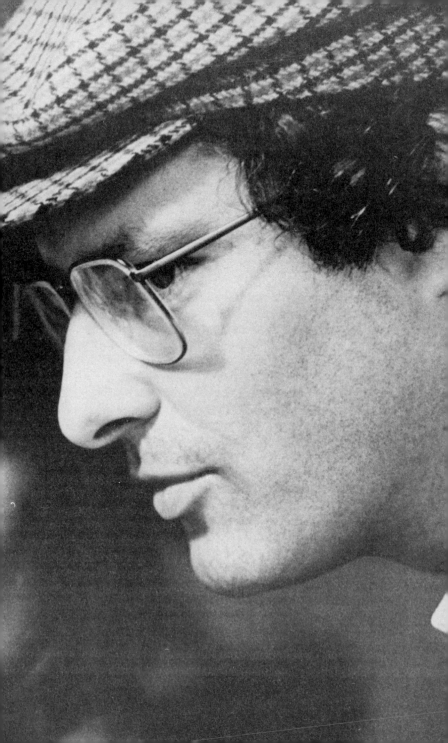

JOHN DUIGAN

John Duigan lives in a comfortably untidy house in the inner Sydney suburb of Rozelle. It's as if his lifestyle, like his politics, has evolved from his student days; there appears to have been no major rupture propelling him into bourgeois luxury or show-business flamboyance. You get the impression that Duigan's sentences are fully formed before he begins the first words. He speaks with deliberation, and there are often lengthy hesitations while he determines exactly what he wants to say next. Several of the directors in this book describe themselves as addicted to or obsessed with filmmaking, and they can have an almost manic quality which corresponds to the magnetism they command. John Duigan gives a different impression: he is a biggish man, but neither his bulk nor his relative success make him the inevitable centre of attention in a room. He has a dry sense of humour and a rather surprised sounding laugh which occasionally interrupts the considered flow of his conversation.

Duigan describes himself as a political filmmaker. His politics are based on a commitment formed in the sixties, a time of ferment and questioning in all areas but one: the moral certainty that the established system was wrong in fighting the war in Vietnam. For Duigan, unlike many veterans of the anti-war movement, the broadly based radicalism of those years was not a phase to be grown through. While words like 'didactic' or 'propagandist' cause some directors to fall back with the sort of horror a vampire displays at the sign of the cross, for John Duigan they simply describe an unsuccessful strategy: a film perceived as didactic is less effective than one whose message is received through its power to move and to entertain.

Duigan's first feature, *The Trespassers* (1976), focused on tensions, attractions and shifting sexual loyalties between a couple, one of whom is in favour of monogamy while the other expresses his disfavour by secretly sleeping around, and a non-possessive young woman who befriends them both. What people do, and what they do to each other, have been central concerns in all John Duigan's films. That is a reflection not just of tactics or philosophy, but of a literary bent – his first adult ambition was to be a writer and he has published one novel – and of a strong interest in performance and character that began with his work in live theatre. Theatre in the late sixties and early seventies was the cutting edge of Australian culture, and the beginning of the alternative theatre boom coincided with John Duigan's arrival at university in 1968. A large part of the next five years he spent working as an actor, and occasionally as a director in student theatre and at La Mama and the Pram Factory, the theatres of Carlton.

Duigan's empathy with actors is evident in his ability to elicit powerful performances from inexperienced actors. In *Mouth to Mouth* (1978), a convincing and entertaining story about four unemployed teenagers, two of his leads had never acted before. He enjoys working with novices: none of the four principals in the 1984 *One Night Stand* are professional performers. He is effective too with experienced actors. In *Winter of our Dreams* (1980), Duigan directed Judy Davis in what is certainly one of her best performances to date, as the King's Cross prostitute, Lou. 'It is important for actors to feel that they are as much a part of the process as the director or the cameraman,' Davis told *Cinema Papers* in 1981. 'John is exceptionally receptive to that way of thinking. On *Winter of our Dreams* I learnt not to be so introverted. There was real trust and that's terribly important for film work.'

John Duigan's politics are underpinned by a characteristically consistent philosophical framework. Existentialism, which emphasises each individual's responsibility for her or his choices, had a profound impact on many young radicals of the sixties. For John Duigan it provided a way of connecting action in the personal and the political spheres that is reflected in all his work. His focus is on individuals, on characters, both in the creation and unfolding of a story and in his vision of how politics is made real.

In 1979 Duigan directed *Dimboola*; he collaborated with the playwright Jack Hibberd on the screenplay. It was an unusual arrangement for Duigan: he is one of a very small number of Australian directors who are sole authors of the films they direct.

Given his background it's probably not surprising that his next film, *Winter of our Dreams* is one of Duigan's most successful films. The principal male character, played by Bryan Brown, is a former sixties activist whose life has lost its excitement and its sense of purpose, and the film directly addresses the interaction between the political, personal and sexual choices people make. Duigan's next film was *Far East*, released in 1982. A romantic adventure with echoes of *Casablanca*, it sought to expose oppression and corruption in the Philippines and the complicity of Australian companies and individuals. *Far East*, like *Winter of our Dreams* and *One Night Stand*, was produced by Richard Mason, an experienced producer remembered by Peter Weir as one of his mentors at the Commonwealth Film Unit.

It's a little disconcerting to find that John Duigan comes from an armed-services background. There is some irony that the writer/director of the anti-nuclear film *One Night Stand* should have among his earliest memories the thrill of watching Britain's nuclear-armed airplanes taking off and landing, and that his father should later have headed a civil defence program in Australia.

Duigan made only minor changes to the interview transcript, but several weeks after approving the final version he telephoned. A critical review of *Far East* had reappeared in the *Sydney Morning Herald*, coinciding with the film's first run on television. Duigan had been stung – could he add an extra paragraph? The desire to answer critical attacks must be a strong one for all directors. Although most affirm that they are immune, there is often an edge in the voice and surprisingly accurate recall of places, names and views expressed in articles about their work. Ingmar Bergman is reported to have once slapped a critic whose review offended him; John Duigan has been satisfied with a written rejoinder, which forms part of the *Far East* discussion below.

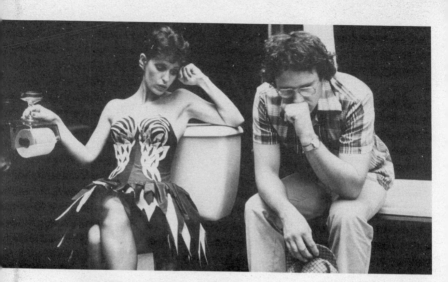

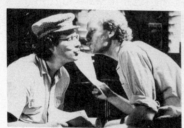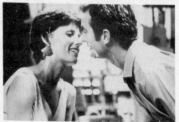

Above: 'I still have ambivalent feelings about some of the costumes.' Helen Morse and John Duigan on the set of *Far East*.

Below left: John Duigan and Michael Falloon (first assistant director) rehearsing for . . .
Below right: Helen Morse (Jo Reeves) and Bryan Brown (Morgan Keefe)'s first kiss in *Far East*.

Right: Judy Davis as the Kings Cross prostitute Lou in *Winter of our Dreams*.

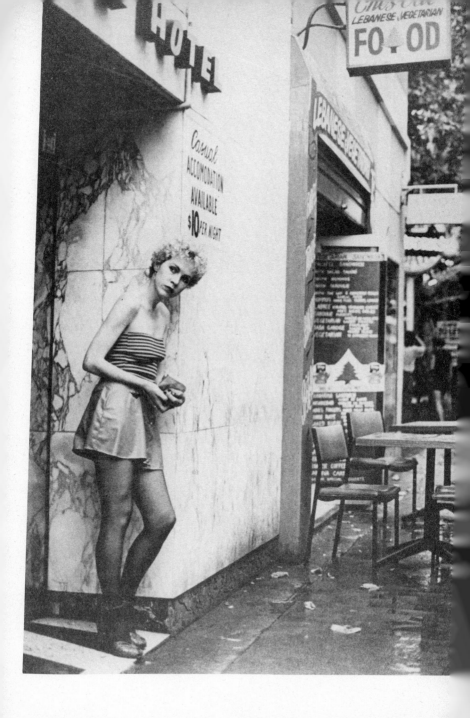

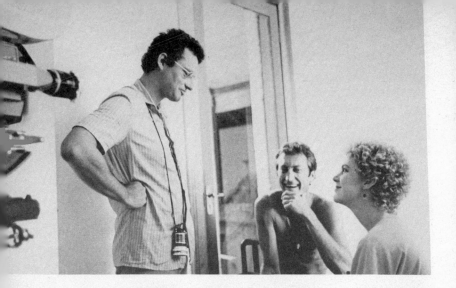

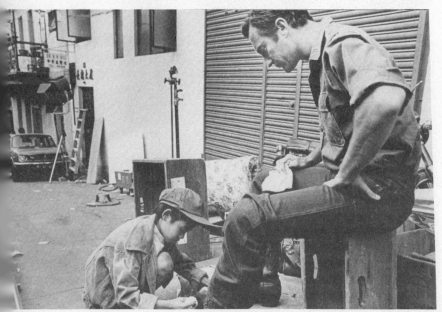

Above: 'Working with actors is one of the most rewarding parts of the whole filmmaking process for me.' John Duigan, Judy Davis and Bryan Brown in *Winter of our Dreams*.

Below: 'Using simple images doesn't involve talking down to an audience.' Bryan Brown (Morgan Keefe) and Sanh Lee Duc (Kip) in *Far East*.

BEGINNINGS

Against the Cringe: Theatre in Carlton

Sue Mathews: Why did you find yourself drawn to the alternative theatre?
John Duigan: I can clearly remember the first time I went to La Mama in Carlton, early in 1969 – it was such an exciting experience. The name La Mama was taken from the New York theatre of the same name and it was started by Betty Burstall, who was then married to the filmmaker Tim Burstall. The theatre was (and still is) in a small warehouse in Carlton. It was a very wet night and there was a fire burning and about thirty people sitting around a small performance area – the play took place in an almost confrontational relationship to the audience, because they were literally inches away. I'd never seen anything like it and found it absolutely thrilling.

Soon after I began to get involved in things like the improvisational activities at La Mama. On weekends three actors would come downstairs, the audience would give them a word and the actors would have one minute to work out a half-hour improvisation based on that word. Improvising for an audience in that kind of situation is probably the most testing and frightening thing an actor can do – a lot of the improvisations were awful but occasionally something very interesting would happen.

It was such a productive and fascinating time, that period at the end of the 1960s. Vietnam meant that an atmosphere of polarisation was growing right through society: there was the interest in Eastern metaphysics; the hippy movement was sweeping in; there were the seeds of the feminist movement; new attitudes to homosexuality; and a much more active confrontation with all sorts of radical political ideas. All of those things provided a very rich environment, out of which came the resurgence of the Australian theatre. The core of that revival in Melbourne was initially at La Mama – it preceded the corresponding rise of the Nimrod in Sydney by a couple of years I think.

*Do you see any links between that theatre revival in Melbourne
and the way the cinema has developed?*
Yes, definitely. There are a number of actors from that period who
have become significant members of the film community – Graeme
Blundell, Bruce Spence, Max Gillies, and Peter Cummins for
instance. Of the directors, Linzee Smith has become quite a prolific
maker of 8mm films in New York, and Alan Finney has a key role as a
marketing director with the exhibitor-distributor Village-Roadshow,
where he's had a sustaining interest in supporting Australian films.
And the writers David Williamson, John Romeril, and Jack Hibberd
have all continued to flourish.

What sorts of things were happening in the alternative theatre?
The majority of writers were trying to create a popular theatre that
would reach a much broader audience than the established
Melbourne Theatre Company and St Martins. There was much
reading of the *Translantic Drama Review* and we would discuss the
plays of the Living Theatre though few of us had seen them. There
was a great stress on making theatre relevant and accessible to the
widest possible audience and that was extended to embrace the idea of
moving out of established theatres. We did a lot of street theatre and
put on plays at factories and work sites, often in conjunction with the
Amalgamated Metal Workers Union, as it was then called. Specific
plays would be written for demonstrations about conditions in
Housing Commission flats, the Vietnam moratoriums, and all sorts of
other issues.
    There was one play we put on to challenge the censorship laws,
called *Whatever Happened to Realism,* following the prosecution of
the actors and director of *Norm and Ahmed,* Alex Buzo's first play.
John Romeril wrote *Whatever Happened to Realism* as a deliberate
challenge to the laws relating to the use of 'foul' language and the
play climaxed with the whole cast singing 'shit, fuck, cunt, fart,
bugger off will you' repeatedly. The play was performed outside La
Mama for three nights until the police came along and arrested the
entire cast and we were taken down to the Carlton Watchhouse, with
about three hundred people from the audience following, also
chanting the song. I can remember being in the cell, hearing the
police ring up, urgently requesting reinforcements because they

thought there was going to be a riot and the crowd might storm the
watchhouse.

How conscious was the nationalism of the alternative theatre?
It was very important. I think the writers Jack Hibberd, John Romeril,
and later on David Williamson, the La Mama directors Alan Finney,
Brian Davies, and Graeme Blundell, and the actors were all very
conscious of the anomaly of Australians having no real models of
themselves to look to. They recognised theatre's role in reflecting
social contradictions and distilling a sense of Australian nationality
and what it is to be an Australian, and a lot of the material certainly
reflected those preoccupations.

Early   Years – From   Drill   to   Drama

You spent your early years outside Australia, didn't you?
Yes. My father was an Australian in the Royal Air Force and my
mother is English; she had been in the WAAF and met my father
during the war. I lived in England until I was ten, and then my father
was transferred to the Royal Malayan Air Force and we lived near
Kuala Lumpur at the airport. After a year and a half there I was sent to
boarding school in Australia. It was the same school my father and
various other Duigans had been to, Geelong College, which is not to
be confused with Geelong Grammar School where Prince Charles
went.

What was boarding school like?
I hated it. I had a pronounced English accent which, for the first
couple of years at least, made me something of a social leper. The
school in many ways resembled the school in Lindsay Anderson's film
If – you got caned repeatedly, there were cold showers in the morning
and persecution by fellow pupils was carried to a fine art. I'm sure
some people were scarred for life by the experiences they went
through there, although arguably it drove people into being able to
cope in public situations – which has its positive and negative sides. It
was an all-male school of course and that tended to increase the
pressure-cooker effect: it was a seething hotbed of frustration! I spent

a lot of my spare time trying to master Australian Rules football, which was totally different from the rugby and soccer I'd played in England and Malaya. It was very important to be at least competent at sport – if you were good, you could transcend anything, even an extreme English accent, but if you were hopeless there was a whole extra area for attack and ridicule. It took me some years before I was able to kick and mark the ball without bringing a derisive jeer from whoever I was attempting to kick it to.

It seems a very English upper-class tradition to send you to the same school as your father.
It was probably more a service tradition. I lived on aerodromes from when I was three until I was eleven and that is a very special kind of lifestyle. It is isolated from the rest of the population, you mix almost exclusively with children of other people from the Air Force, and in a way all Air Force children felt that civilians from outside were in some way inferior. For three years we lived on RAF Scampton which is one of the bases where the V bombers, which for many years were the main thrust of Britain's nuclear deterrent force, were based, and we would go up to the runway and watch these huge delta-shaped white aeroplanes taking off around dusk. They were constantly out on patrol with nuclear weapons on board – of course in those days, I simply saw them as vast, incredibly noisy but very beautiful aeroplanes. To a kid who plays with toy soldiers and model planes, the service lifestyle seems quite exciting and in fact my ambitions were to become either a marshal of the Royal Air Force or an admiral of the Fleet, until my first day in cadets at Geelong College: I found to my horror that military discipline, having to clean brass and boots and perform ludicrous forms of drill in an obsessive manner were the last things I was interested in doing. So all those ambitions went down to the bottom rung completely and my next ambition, which was to be a writer, came to the top.

Having spent your early childhood outside Australia you probably didn't share the cultural cringe of many Australian kids of the fifties.
I really had a fairly positive and romantic view of Australia, gained through books that my father's relations would send over for

Christmas – books like *The Magic Pudding, Aboriginal Legendary Tales,* and *Blinky Bill.* I was genuinely looking forward to coming out here – Australia seemed like a pretty exciting sort of place.

Did you read a lot, or were you a TV child?
I was a prolific reader. I used to read volumes of military history as well as the usual childrens' books of the fifties like *Biggles* and *The Famous Five.* Reading was much more important for me as a kid than watching television. It must have been 1954 when we got television, because I can remember going down to a neighbour's house to watch the coronation in 1953. There were a number of series I liked a lot – the original *Robin Hood* series, with Richard Greene; *Boots and Saddles,* about the Fifth Cavalry; and there was a comedy called *The Army Game* I used to like.

Where you much aware of American culture?
The main American influence came from television. America was scarcely studied at all at school in Australia; British history was what I studied in my senior years. But in my first year at boarding school, on Saturday nights we would watch *Leave It to Beaver, Disneyland* and *Rawhide,* which of course are three American television shows. We would buy bottles of soft drink and maybe threepence worth of chips and sit up in our pyjamas and dressing gowns watching these shows before going to bed – you'd put holes in the tops of the bottles with compasses so you could suck the Tarax Pine or Tarax Crimson out very slowly and make it last the full two and a half hours.

Were you interested in movies as a kid?
I always liked films very much and have quite a detailed recall of films that were important to me. When I lived in England my favourites were films on military subjects, like *Reach for the Sky, The Dambusters,* and an American film that I particularly liked called *Away All Boats.* Another film that left an inordinate impression was *The Forbidden Planet,* a marvellous science-fiction film which completely terrified me, and when I lived in Malaya I saw *Ben Hur* and *Psycho* – that certainly terrified me as well.

I didn't see many films while I was at boarding school, but I can remember in my final year saving up my money and taking my then

girlfriend from our sister school up to Melbourne on the train to see
Who's Afraid of Virginia Woolf? I'd hoped it would be something of a
turn on, but in fact the film completely obliterated any thoughts of
cuddling; it was so unrelievedly heavy we could barely speak to each
other for the rest of the day and returned sitting side by side on the
train to Geelong in a kind of numb state.

Was it a shock to go straight from school to university?
No, it was exhilarating. I couldn't wait to get out of school: I was
terrifically excited about going to university and I found it to be right
up to my expectations. I'd had six years of increasingly bitter
relations with the teachers at school and in the early years bitter
relations with a lot of the other kids. I found the whole structure of
rules and regulations almost unbearable, so university was an
incredible burst of freedom. I lived in a state of high excitement at
university for the first few years I was there.

What were you studying?
My parents persuaded me to do Law on the grounds that a writer
should have something to fall back on. The first cases they set you I'm
sure were the most lurid they could pick, to lead you into the
misapprehension that Law was going to be titillating – the legal
implications of people starving on a rowing boat and eating one
another, that kind of thing. But I quickly realised they were not in the
least representative of what was in store and I managed to transfer to
Arts part way through the first year and studied Philosophy and
History instead. I did a Masters in Philosophy, with a thesis entitled *A
Sketch Towards a Humanistic Theory of Ethics.* My main interests
were ethics, political philosophy, and contemporary European
philosophy, particularly existentialism. The Melbourne University
philosophy department was strongest in the fields of logic and the
philosophy of language, but I found both these areas arid and
removed – I was much more interested in philosophy that I felt
engaged with life in the wider world.

*Were you engaged with the wider issues of the time – the anti-war
movement for example?*
Yes – I would speak at meetings, and I was often involved in street

theatre shows about the war and conscription. I became active in
theatre quite early on and that became my main area of activity – in
fact I spent more time working in theatre than on my course. I worked
with a university theatre group at first, then I got involved at La Mama
and became a member of the Australian Performing Group when it
first formed.

The Search for an Audience

*Were you aware during this very active theatre period of a move to
start making movies?*
Not really, no. What happened was that while I was working as an
actor in La Mama I was seen by some of the filmmakers in Carlton and
I was cast in some of their films. There was a nucleus of people who
had come from the film society at Melbourne University. Some of
these people were actively involved in La Mama itself, and others
would often go and see plays there, so it was natural that many of the
films would use La Mama actors. Tim Burstall used Bruce Spence for
Stork after seeing him in plays at La Mama, Brian Davies cast me as
the lead in his film *Brake Fluid*, then Nigel Buesst cast me in *Bonjour
Balwyn*. *Brake Fluid* won a national award, but the announcement
was booed by the Sydney audience – they thought Peter Weir's
Homesdale should have won.

*Were you aware of the pressure that some people were then
putting on the government to allocate funds to support an
Australian film industry?*
No, I wasn't. But I think that was because at that stage I had no
interest in becoming a filmmaker myself. I still saw myself principally
as an actor and later on as a writer – every now and then I would work
on a novel I was writing called *Badge,* which was later published by
Macmillan. So I was unaware of all the lobbying. I wasn't even
especially conscious of the fledgling film industry and the incredible
difficulties filmmakers were having to get any kinds of films made.
We knew of Tim Burstall as a maker of big films in Carlton and there
was a lot of interest when he made *Stork* – I became aware then that
he had had to do things like mortgage his house to raise money for it. I

knew nothing of the activities of Fred Schepisi and the Producers'
and Directors' Guild.

*Were you familiar with the Australian films of the twenties and
thirties?*
I was not even aware that there had been a film industry here – I had
seen virtually no Australian film at all.

*Both the theatre and the film revivals in Melbourne seem to have
germinated in Carlton – why do you think that was?*
Well, Carlton is and was then even more so a university suburb. An
enormous number of university students lived there, and many of the
people who became important figures in film and theatre came from
the university. Sydney has no corresponding single suburb of
students, and the counter-culture is much more diffuse. The Carlton
background for filmmaking and theatre was very different from any
of the formative processes in Sydney, as it was from other filmmaking
that grew up in Melbourne later on. I think maybe the chief
distinguishing feature was the political environment in which the
theatre and filmmaking arose. It was particularly an aspect of the
theatre scene and it exercised – and continues to exercise –
considerable influence over the people who came out of it.

*When did you begin to consider filmmaking as an activity that
you might want to pursue yourself?*
It was after the second of two six-week tours with the Melbourne
University Student Theatre. We called them the kaleidoscope tours –
we bought an old bus and a blow-up bubble tent, about 60 feet long,
and a group of about 35 of us toured through Gippsland and up the
south coast of New South Wales to Sydney and then back across
inland. It was a fairly major logistical enterprise: we did plays on the
beach, on the street, and at night in church halls, RSL clubs, or
surf-lifesaving clubs. It was all part of the idea of taking theatre to the
people. But at the end of the second tour it became clear to me that the
idea of getting vast new audiences for theatre was stretching things
and that if I was interested in exploring subjects for a wider audience
then film was the medium to go into.

So it was quite a pragmatic decision rather than any sudden

excitement in the process of filmmaking. I started work on a script: this was when the first funding bodies were being set up and because I could list about seven small films in which I'd been an actor and sometimes co-writer, I had a reasonably comprehensive-sounding background on which to move into directing and I was able to get a small grant for *The Firm Man*.

What was The Firm Man *about?*
It was a very ambitious subject, over-complex, and I'm afraid rather opaque as far as the audience is concerned. It was about a man called Gerald, played brilliantly by Peter Cummins, who is working successfully as a businessman for an organisation called Kroop and Kroop. He is approached by an organisation called the Firm which is a transnational organisation of monolithic size – we never get to know much about this organisation and what it does, but it is a glamour organisation and it is very flattering for anyone to be invited to join it. Gerald is put through a series of very perplexing and absurd-seeming exercises and at the same time his marriage is crumbling, and the whole world as he knows it begins to disintegrate. In fact the Firm is behind all this. The film is a study of manipulation and alienation.

So it was an interest in reaching an audience that was the primary factor – what sorts of things did you want to say to them?
I wanted to explore philosophical, political, or psychological subjects generally with an ethical basis to them plus an interest in the exploration of characters. Those have been abiding and continuing interests.

You were more interested in saying things than in performance?
No, I would say that I was equally interested in both those things. What I wasn't particularly interested in at first was the technical process of filmmaking and the filmmaking medium as such – technical curiosity was not a starting point for me. I learnt about the actual process of filmmaking through making *The Firm Man* and having done that I realised my great technical limitations and spent the next two years watching films in a totally different way. Since

those times, I've become much more interested in the technicalities of filmmaking and evolving a personal style – one of the reasons that I have stayed in filmmaking is that I very rapidly grew to love the medium and the whole process of making a film. But the love affair with filmmaking was a by-product of actually making films rather than a cause of getting involved which I think is probably unusual.

MAKING   THE   MOVIES

The   Trespassers

The Trespassers *was your first major feature. It was about the shifting relationships between three people, two women and a man, and it raised questions about jealousy and monogamy and couples. You made the film in 1976 but set it in 1970 – why didn't you set it in the present?*
I wanted to contrast the behaviour of the characters in their private lives with their wider political lives, because in many ways there was a major discrepancy between them. Their socio-political activities and beliefs were generally admirable but their personal politics were in a state of extreme confusion. 1970 was the time of maximum awareness of Vietnam and conscription and just preceded the impact of feminism in Australia – it is a particular, very distinct period, with very distinct speech rhythms and language. One thing I forgot to mention when I was talking about the nexus of influences that coincided in the late sixties was of course the sexual revolution; it swamped Melbourne University like a tidal wave in 1967-68, my first two years there. It threw interaction between men and women, women and women, and men and men into a heightened and very different state of affairs from the years preceding and following it. So *The Trespassers* reflects the characters' and my own grapplings with some of the implications of that. We were still grappling with them in 1976.

The Trespassers *shares a very intense interest in those personal issues with Helen Garner's novel* Monkey Grip, *which also came from the place and period in which you made the film. Why do you think people were so concerned with those questions in the middle seventies?*

Those things were raised at the turn of the decade and we were evaluating them and analysing them more critically by the middle seventies. I don't think at first we realised the full implications of the whole way our lifestyles were changing – questions were raised of such a fundamental nature about the way we relate to our friends and partners, and those questions are much more immediate than any other kind. They are certainly more tangible and closer to home than questions of a wider political kind, so I think it is inevitable that we would start addressing ourselves to them collectively. I'm talking in the main about that group who were educated in the late sixties and early seventies –echoes from that period have now gone out to the rest of society, but essentially it began in that group. Another reason for that period of assessment was that we were five years older and people who had been 17 to 21 at the end of the sixties were now starting to think about settling down and having to make choices about getting married and raising families or opting to continue with an alternative way of relating to people. Also of course that early period was so frenetic that one didn't have much time for thinking, one was too busy rushing about participating in it and doing it.

After The Trespassers *what happened?*

I took *The Trespassers* to the Cannes Film Festival. I was completely broke when I got back and I took a job at the Royal Melbourne Institute of Technology, RMIT, directing educational documentaries on building a bridge and metal finishing. I was also working on the script of *Mouth to Mouth* and trying to get money for that. Then they gave me the job of trying to put the fledgling radio station 3RRR on a financial footing and I spent the next few months attending committee meetings. I wasn't able really to do much on the creative side of the radio station because it was a full-time job just getting the thing backed by enough people in the RMIT to keep it going, and sustaining the balancing act necessary between the radio station itself and the students who also worked on it. Around this time the money came through for *Mouth to Mouth* – after three refusals the Victorian Film Corporation finally agreed to support it – and as I had already worked three months over my six months contract, I left to do *Mouth to Mouth.*

Were you doing pre-production at the same time as trying to run the radio station?
No. What I did do was look around for my cast and I did find one of the cast working at the RMIT as a van driver. I used him to play a caveman in the metal finishing film – I was trying to put some comedy into the film to keep the students who would have to sit through it awake. So I had things like a bath scene with him and an old girlfriend of mine (which had to be drastically cut), and a scene where he discovers metal for the first time when he sets some ore-bearing rock around his camp fire and in the morning he finds a small deposit of melted metal and grunts at it. His name was Serge Frazzetto and I cast him as one of the four leads in *Mouth to Mouth.*

M o u t h   t o   M o u t h

There seems to be a quantum leap between The Trespassers *and* Mouth to Mouth – *what does that reflect?*
The single main thing was that I decided that I didn't really like *The Trespassers* as a film and why I didn't like it was that I hadn't written enough humour or warmth into the characters, they weren't engaging. The film in part was about people rationalising the world to death, analysing things to the point of torturing themselves and squeezing all spontaneity out, so they had to be like that, but it meant it was a film you might respect rather than like. I wanted to make a film where the characters were much more sympathetic and accessible and who related to the world from an immediate and spontaneous point of view.

Why a story about unemployed kids? At least on the surface it seems quite a long way removed from your own life.
Living in an inner-city suburb the unemployment problem was beginning to become visible in 1977-78 and I thought it was a problem that needed talking about – in those days it hadn't become the

much-discussed issue it is these days. There was very little awareness of it but there were still homeless kids living around the inner suburbs of Australian cities, that was the motivation for doing it.

What sort of research did you do? Did you talk to kids in that situation?
I knew social workers who worked with unemployed people and I had friends who were unemployed. I did spend time at Winlaton, the state detention and training centre for adolescent girls – some of the girls read the script and we talked about it at some length. The two actresses spent a day there and we did a bit of shooting there too. I also had a friend in my early days at university who had been at Turana, the equivalent boys home, and we had done some of our student plays out at Turana so that was another kind of link.

The dialogue and the manners and the ways the kids behave with each other seems very accurate, very right, so I'm surprised that you didn't do much in terms of talking to people like them.
They are typical of a much larger group than simply people who are unemployed or have been in social welfare institutions: they are typical working-class teenagers. Two of the actors, Serge and Sonia Peat, came roughly from those sorts of backgrounds, and the other two, who had some experience of acting, were both very good actors. All four of them put in terrific performances.

Did that create any difficulties, having two of your principal cast who were experienced and two who were not?
No, because they all got on well – we spent a week away together rehearsing at a house on the beach which was very helpful because we all got to know each other. It was really rehearsed in great detail: there was no improvisation, and the script didn't change much during the rehearsal period so we were able to concentrate on the text and getting the performances right. I like to have at least a two-week rehearsal period with all the films I do, ideally three weeks.

The unemployment issue is nicely integrated, punctuating the film with the scenes at the factory and the dole office. How did

*you conceive the relationship between the social and political
points you wanted to make and the story?*

I started off with the four characters and built up their interaction. In
general that's how I've tended to write all my films – the characters
precede the plot. The things I wanted to explore in it –the sexual role
interplay, the issues of unemployment and growing alienation, the
impact that situation has on their choices about petty theft and going
into prostitution – all those elements came in reasonably organically
from the starting point of the characters. One of the interesting
dynamics in the characters is that the two boys come from the country
and the two girls from social welfare institutions. The girls are in
many ways much more worldly than the guys, and a lot of the decision
making and impetus comes from them, but that is balanced by the fact
that the guys have a more developed moral perspective. That meant
that sometimes there was a wider sort of evaluation between the four,
because they bring different ingredients into their relationships.

How happy do you feel with it looking back at it now?

I feel very happy with *Mouth to Mouth*. I was very confident during
the making of it, I felt that it was the right cast and it was a good
shoot, with no major problems in it. It was very tight – we had just
four weeks, using a small crew, and almost all the locations were very
close together. The production office organised the whole thing
extremely well and the thing came in – there are very few things I'd
change in it.

*The director of photography was Tom Cowan – was it the first
time you'd worked together?*

We'd worked together when I'd been acting in *Bonjour Balwyn* back
in 1971. I'd liked his work since so I approached him and it turned out
very well. We enjoy working together. He is an enormously tranquil
person in himself and that is a very useful and rare quality to have in a
person on a film crew because it produces a very calming, stabilising
effect. Particularly in the position of d.o.p., because the cameraman is
so central on the crew: the equipment and the technicians revolve
around the camera – it is a sort of altar in a way.

Dimboola

Dimboola *was based on the Jack Hibberd play about a country
wedding. It is the one film you didn't write as well as direct and I
gather that was not an altogether happy arrangement.*
No, Jack Hibberd, who wrote the original very successful play, and I
were never really able to come to complete agreement about the
script. We had ultimately different conceptions of it – he conceived
it as much more robust and ribald, while I wanted something gentler
and more lyrical and the two points of view created a tension in the
film that lessened its overall coherence. However, the major
pressure on the film was that it was an extremely complicated film,
but we only had a very small budget and had to shoot it in five
weeks. I think it was just impossible to do justice to it in five weeks
– it was a week longer than, say, the *Mouth to Mouth* shoot but
logistically *Mouth to Mouth* was a much simpler canvas whereas
Dimboola was a great big sprawling film with about thirty or forty
central characters. It meant we were never able to do as much
coverage as I would have liked – we constantly had to simplify
scenes and rush them through and I don't think we were even able
to do enough work with the cast.

Even so I think there are some good things about the film and there
is one particular scene which is almost my favourite scene from any of
the films I've directed. It is the scene where the Max Gillies character
cycles into the town at night and goes to listen to three girls, the
Milkshakes, rehearsing their annual musical, and then wanders out
and climbs up the stairs of the pub to his room. The camera cranes up
and he appears in silhouette and lights his pipe then pulls up the blind
and blows a draught of smoke out into the cold night air – I was
particularly happy with that scene.

How did you feel about the critical reaction to Dimboola?
I felt it suffered an unwarranted drubbing. It came out at a stage when
the critics were wanting some serious examinations of the Australian
character that went beyond the 'nasty, brutish and short' ocker
version of Australian life, and so they were much more damning of the
film than perhaps they would have been had it come out a year or two
earlier or later. It is really quite an affectionate film that celebrates

people living in a country town; it is not a particularly gross or even caricaturish look at them. The bucks' turn for example was very mild compared to some of the stories we were told by the locals at Dimboola itself where the film was shot – we could have had much more grotesque things happening. So there was no real attempt to see what else was being said in the film – there were some quite nice little moral tales between some of the characters, there was a lot of humour and warmth, and there were some good performances the critics chose not to see.

Winter   of   our   Dreams

In Winter of our Dreams, *the principal male character, Rob, has been prompted by the suicide of a friend, Lisa, to write an article about what happened to the radicals of the sixties. Is that a question that was of major concern for you, as it was for him?*
Well for him it's a sort of attempt to chart a spiritual decline. I don't think he would rationally see it like that but I think that unconsciously that is what it is for him. I think it is an important subject but I would tackle it in a slightly different way, namely by doing *Winter.*

Was it a question that preoccupied you?
Yes, but it is part of a wider question. The film is an attempt to examine the prevailing mood at the early stages of the eighties and to explore what happened during the seventies to some people who were radicals in the late sixties. They represent a much wider cross-section of society than the comparatively few who like Rob and his wife Gretel were university educated. In contrast, the character of Lou comes from the middle seventies in terms of her formative period. She is someone who has no real perception of political or sociological or philosophical problems as such.

The Rob character in my background material had come from a working-class background and had opted for a middle-class lifestyle. We see photographs and hear descriptions of him in Lisa's diary that showed him to be an inspiring firebrand at university but there is very little of that remaining in the character we see playing chess with a machine in the bookshop and confronting his moral dilemmas through exhaustive rational analysis. Rob's life is contrasted with Lou's more razor-edge existence. Lou is someone whose sense of self is a fluctuating unity of disparate bits and pieces of behaviour that have impressed her from other people she has seen. She responds to the world in an immediate sense and she gets damaged very easily. Her responses to problems occur through quite different processes to Rob's and I think that the contrast between these rational and intuitive ways of being-in-the-world was maybe for me the central element of the film.

You said in an interview with Cinema Papers *that meeting Lou reminds Rob of a more emotional, intuitive part of himself that was more prominent in the sixties. I wondered if you meant that to apply to his relationships and particularly to his relationship with Lisa, because the film struck me as a study of a man who has not been able to respond directly or honestly to women. Particularly with regard to his treatment of Lisa and Lou, it struck me as a study in bad faith and I doubted whether Rob was really more emotional and intuitive in those earlier days.*

In his dealings with Lisa he appears to have behaved, according to the diary entries, in similar ways that he behaves towards Lou, and there is a sense of repetition. The title that I wanted to give the film was *Deja Vu*, which relates to that and to the way that the relationship with Lou seems to inexorably follow the pattern of the earlier relationship. But I don't see the Rob character as dishonest. I think what you say about bad faith is an interesting reading of the film but I see Rob as paradoxically being quite a profoundly honest person and I think he has always attempted to deal honestly with the people he has been close to.

He is always stressing the need for people to take responsibility for what they do which is a very central ethical principle in my opinion – for example, in the scene where Lou is attempting to impress him with her lurid junkie's description of the danger, risk, and glamour of living on the razor's edge, he'll have nothing of that and really belittles her story about the guy injecting into a vein in his eye. He tells her quite categorically that it is her decision to get off the stuff and his behaviour to Lou throughout is quite consistent with that.

I think you can read the diary entries of his relationship with Lisa as having a similar kind of consistency: he realised how much he meant to her and how his making love to her would be of overwhelming significance to this very romantic and vulnerable person. So he tried to belittle the sexual side of their relationship – he says to her in the diary 'there you are, it wasn't such a big deal, was it?' It is an attempt, in the same way that he treats Lou, to try and stress to the person 'don't build up your expectations about me, don't come to rely on me or look for any enduring relationship because that is not what I want or feel able to give to you.' However at the end of the film when we have watched Rob remaining aloof from Lou as she is almost disintegrating in front of him, we see him in the football sheds going through a crisis that is really about the way he has chosen to live his life. The analytical approach he embraced in the late sixties and that he has remained consistent with have somehow cut out some fundamental aspect of living.

That's quite a different view of Rob from the one I got. I saw him very much as someone who was prepared to accept affection but not take responsibility for that. He is ambiguous with Lou a lot of the time – for instance, in the last encounter between Rob and Lou she says 'it's no good, is it?' and he says 'what isn't?' as though he really doesn't understand that she is referring to the possibility of a relationship with him. How did you intend that?

He is trying to pretend that he really doesn't know that she thinks that much of him, that she is expecting or hoping for some kind of relationship, in order to stress to her that he has no expectations at all in that direction.

Why can't he say that – why does he pretend that he doesn't understand? By pretending not to understand he sustains the illusion of possibility . . .

Yes, he probably does do that and can be criticised for that but what he is feeling is that he wants her to find that path herself, to arrive at a point where she says 'God, I don't want to have anything to do with this person' – he wants her to make that leap for her own good.

It's a fairly unrealistic hope, that two people will agree precisely about the appropriateness or inappropriateness of a relationship at exactly the same time.

That is the sort of thing the film is getting at – you can rationalise the world to a point where you lose touch with reality and that is what has happened to Rob, that is what his tragedy is. So it is a different kind of problem from bad faith, but maybe a really central one with many people.

How do you see Rob's relationship with his wife, Gretel? Do you think that is so rationalised as to have lost its reality?

Well they share the same starting points in their values and their ways of being-in-the-world, so their relationship doesn't suffer from the same kind of contradictions. In its own terms it's not a bad relationship. It is refreshingly honest, and I think there is genuine love and affection and humour there, but it lacks the dimension that Rob becomes intuitively aware of in the football sheds. So it is basically impoverished.

You describe Rob and Gretel's relationship as 'refreshingly honest' and yet the degree to which it is honest has to do with the degree to which it is highly rationalised, in the much-discussed agreement that both of them can have affairs.

Yes. Some people would argue that their need for affairs is a grasping out for something that is lacking in their own relationship or a sign of immaturity. That might be true to the extent that their relating to other people comes from the sense that it is the appropriate way of living and that something is wrong if one or other of them doesn't, rather than from being genuinely attracted to someone else. In so far as it is that, yes, it is a product of the rationalising-to-death syndrome but I don't for one minute want to be seen to be saying in the film that the desire or attraction one feels for other people from time to time and the decision to act on that is immature or irreconcilable with a fully mature relationship.

There is a clear contrast in the film between Rob and Gretel's house and the world that Lou occupies.

Yes. It's heightened by the way the camera is used in the two worlds –

Lou's world is much more frenetic, there are many more shots, and
the pace of the cutting is more jagged. In Rob and Gretel's house the
style is much more graceful, fluid, and languorous, there are long
tracking shots – some people would say more sterile, though I
wouldn't say that.

*Is there criticism implied in the depiction of Rob and Gretel's
world?*
I am very critical of them. I feel that people who have had the
opportunities they have had, have more of a responsibility to
contribute to society's evolution than they accept. They have really
opted out. I think a lot of people who are like Rob and Gretel have
become very cynical about the possibility of change from the grass
roots and that contributes to spiritual lethargy and pessimism, which
is very obvious in Rob.

I think optimism is incredibly important and one of the good things
about the sixties was how optimistic that time was. The final image of
the film is of the anti-nuclear protestors, who, however doubtful you
might be of their effectiveness, nonetheless do think enough about
the issues to actually go there and make that statement. And the
action of making that statement is vital for people and a society.

*Do you identify Rob and Gretel's choice of a nice house in
Balmain and the bourgeois trimmings of their life with the
disappearance of any kind of commitment and optimism?*
Only superficially. I don't think one has to live in squats to contribute
effectively to political change.

*What drew you to cast Bryan Brown? He is known for much more
broadly drawn, almost ocker characterisations, for example in*
Breaker Morant *or* A Town Like Alice, *than for portrayals of the
more complex characters you tend to write.*
Bryan himself was at university in the late sixties and he shares the
left-wing political stance of a character like Rob, so he has a lot of
experience to draw on when playing the character. Secondly he is a
highly energised individual. Giving him a character in which his own
personal energy is repressed created an emotional reservoir which
made it believable that he could have been an inspiring firebrand

leader in the late sixties. The character is in many ways an infuriating one and you suspect there is another kind of person boiling away somewhere inside.

You used him again in Far East *– you are obviously drawn to him as an actor.*
Yes, I think he is a fine actor and I enjoyed working with him on *Winter* – he is someone who takes acting very seriously. In casting Bryan in *Far East,* I was using much more of his natural character than I was with Rob – Bryan is much closer to Morgan Keefe than he is to Rob McGregor. People talk about him being archetypically Australian and that is an important resource in him. In *Winter* I hoped the inner tension created by having him play a character who on the surface is so different would be very strong for the film and I think it proved to be the case. I was very happy with all the perfomances in *Winter* – Bryan's character is not about emotions, it is about the repression of emotions so of course it goes without saying that it doesn't have the emotional range that is demanded of the actress who is playing Lou.

Was Judy Davis your first choice for the part of Lou?
Yes, she was. I had seen her in *My Brilliant Career* and liked her a lot. Then I saw her in the television series *Water Under the Bridge* and there were a couple of things she did in that role that made me determined to approach her for *Winter of our Dreams.* The characters she played in those other two projects were completely different from Lou – I think both Judy and Bryan were attracted to the roles partly because they were so completely different from any they had done before.

Judy actually spent time in Kings Cross, Sydney's red-light district, in preparation for playing Lou, who is a prostitute, didn't she?
Yes, she moved into Kings Cross about three weeks before the shoot and stayed there during the filming. She has in fact since bought a house in that area. She spent a lot of time wandering around the Cross at night, and occasionally during the rehearsal period I spent time doing that with her. She met a number of prostitutes and spent

evenings talking with them and watched one of them shooting up and
preparing her kit and that kind of thing. She does a great deal of
preparation.

*Did she discover things that surprised you? Did you do as much
research as she did?*
I did a lot of research on the character and the character's
background. I think the sorts of areas that she would bring in
addition to that were particular ways of expressing the psychological
reality of the character and, for example, elements of the way the
character moved.

Far East

Far East *seemed to come out a lot more quickly than* Winter of our
Dreams – *was it produced in more of a hurry?*
No, I think they had about the same time scale. What happened was
that between *Dimboola* and *Winter of our Dreams* I wrote huge
numbers of drafts for a script that I couldn't get the money for. It was
called *Deja Vu,* the name I'd wanted to use for *Winter.* It was about a
girl who had been involved with the Baader-Meinhof group in
Germany. Her boyfriend had been killed when a bomb that he'd
planted exploded prematurely. She'd come to Australia with a small
child, under a false passport, and she develops a relationship with a
disc jockey of a fairly highbrow jazz program. The main character
had become disenchanted with violence as a method of goading
change in contemporary Western societies and was attempting to
come to terms with that, and searching for an alternative.

I just couldn't get the money for it – it was felt to be
'uncommercial'. It's a film I always regret I couldn't get off the
ground, because in its time I think it was important. But when I finally
stopped writing drafts of that I wrote the drafts of *Winter of our
Dreams* in a reasonably short time. In fact the character of Rob was
heavily derived from the male character in *Deja Vu.* I only did about
five or six drafts of *Winter,* whereas I think I did 23 drafts of *Deja Vu.*
And there were about six drafts of *Far East.*

Why a film about the Philippines, where did that idea come from?

Richard Mason, the producer, had been in Manila making a film about poverty there and he had met a girl who had spent three years in a military prison. He played me a tape in which the girl described how she had been arrested along with a close girlfriend, and how her friend had been raped and murdered by the military. She described her period in prison and the sorts of things that happened there – it was a fairly graphic and disturbing tape and I decided to do some research with the idea of making a film.

Did you go to Manila yourself at that stage?

I spent several weeks there. I met the girl and various other people, including trade unionists from the alternative trade unions, the genuine trade unions which operate under constant threat and harassment. We talked to people working in the slums: there is a much greater discrepancy between rich and poor than in any other Eastern country I have seen. There is extraordinary wealth in the Philippines, and the poverty is largely blocked from the public view – there are walls built around the slums. The regime appears to be riddled with corruption, and the government is backed by a strong army which maintains order through terror in sections of the countryside. We also saw the presence of Westerners there, Australians in particular, and the multinationals at work. Australians are among the most numerous tourists – there is a thriving girlie bar scene that caters heavily for Australians.

That material provided a backdrop for an attempt to depict Australians in a Third World country – and to glimpse Western cultural and economic exploitation of the Third World. I wanted to make a film that would reach a large mainstream audience, more so than *Winter*. I wanted to reach the sorts of people who go to such countries as tourists in increasingly large numbers, and the business people who have dealings there – that was the intention, more so than reaching audiences already aware of such things.

So the intention and the research preceded the actual story?

Yes. I then tried to come up with a story that would allow something of the situation we saw there to be revealed. At the same time a secondary theme emerged and that was the moral problems encountered by the four principal characters, who are all very different. The character played by Bryan Brown, Morgan Keefe, is a curious pragmatist – he had come from an orphan background and had been to Vietnam with the army. His experience of the world was one of moral chaos and his response to that was to create the Koala Klub, his nightclub, a place that does have a kind of morality, a sort of oasis of personal order within a anarchic world. But the way he runs the place can be severely criticised from other moral perspectives such as that of Peter Reeves, the journalist, played by John Bell. He is a genuinely concerned left-wing journalist, but he is also ambitious and likes the idea of what he is , he likes the romance and adventure.

Between them is the character of Jo Reeves played by Helen Morse. She grew up in what was Indochina, where she became a singer in a nightclub in Saigon. She and the Morgan Keefe character met in those dangerous days when each time you saw someone you knew it might be the last. She shared his view of the world to a certain extent, but then became involved with Peter Reeves and chose to leave the country with him. She now has an ambivalent attitude to the educated, considered social and political views of her husband – on the one hand she is impressed by this disciplined, compassionate view of the world but she retains a residue of affection for her old hedonistic life.

The fourth prinicipal character is Rosita, the Filipino activist, whose life has been a desperate battle with the government as the editor of a small journal that catalogues political arrests and disappearances, and her commitment to her political principles is total, unswerving to the point of a fixation.

As I was writing the script I created a series of similarities with *Casablanca*, an old favourite of mine. I set the initial character dynamic along similar lines, namely a triangular situation, with the female walking into the nightclub with her husband some years after a love affair, to find her old lover running it. From then on the film goes in very different directions, and to me the interest in the contrast with *Casablanca* is in the totally distinct moral problems that the characters face. The moral dilemmas are very much more complex and confused than those faced by Ingrid Bergman and Humphrey Bogart and company. In that situation there was no doubt who was the enemy – it was the Nazis and they were evil without qualification.

There is no such clear cut enemy in *Far East.*

Surely the multinationals are clearly identified as villains?
Yes, there are definitely villains in the multinationals and the soldiers
who do the torturing. But the principal characters are harder to
evaluate – it is difficult not to find Morgan Keefe admirable in some
ways and despicable in others, just as it is hard to work out Peter
Reeves' priorities in his work, and to evaluate Jo's decision to leave
Manila with her husband.

She makes a parallel choice to that made by Ingrid Bergman in
Casablanca, *which is one we admire. But Jo Reeves' choice is not a
moral or political one, it seems to be made on purely personal
grounds.*
Ingrid Bergman doesn't make a choice, she allows Humphrey to
make the choice for her, that is one of the differences between the
films. Jo Reeves makes the decision to leave Morgan Keefe and it *is*
ultimately a moral decision. Because the thing that sways her is the
discovery that to locate her missing husband Morgan Keefe has had
to prostitute the youngest girl in the Koala Klub and that is itself an
extremely difficult moral decision to evaluate. But that reveals to Jo
the extraordinary network of moral balances and counterbalances
and levels of exploitation that are implicit in Morgan Keefe's world
and her decision is finally that she can't be part of that world – I think
if she was making the decision on purely personal grounds she would
have stayed.

I think all the characters go through some sort of moral
development during the film. Morgan Keefe is forced to come out of
that little closed world that he has created for himself. Against his will
and not through any moral insight initially, he is pulled out of it by his
love for this woman. The state of mind in which he makes that final
decision is both mingled anger and despair about Jo and a kind of fury
at himself because he realises that he has constantly refused to face
up to the sort of lifestyle he has opted for, and he does react ultimately
with dignity. But I don't think people find him a hero because of all
those ambiguous elements. It would probably be easier for the
audience to like the film if he was a more pure hero than he is.

How different was the process of writing the script for Far East *from writing* Winter of our Dreams?

I think one of the differences was that I felt I had to write something closer to a genre plot, a thriller plot, to carry the subject matter closer to the audience. Whereas in *Winter*, the plot came simply through the evolution of the characters, the characters did not throw up a complete plot with *Far East*.

I'm interested in your assumption that the wider audience is more comfortable with a genre orienation. What sorts of choices are entailed in making that decision?

It is a genre plot but not wholly a genre film – if the characters were genre characters they would be heroes and villains. Also, Rob, Gretel and Lou in *Winter of our Dreams* are characters from minority groups. Morgan Keefe in *Far East*, while his life has been extraordinarily idiosyncratic, is none the less much more typical of a broader stream of Australian society than the characters in *Winter*. That makes it more appropriate to open up the subject to a wider audience because they have an immediate point of identification. More generally, thinking about that wider audience probably involves attempting to structure a faster pace for the film and to express the substance and subtleties in ways other than dialogue and character nuance.

It may be true that the Morgan Keefe character is closer to the audience, but on another level both he and the character of Jo are far more glamorous and romantic than any others in your films.

That does come from the desire to open the film up to the mainstream cinema-going audience. The characters do have this heightened quality and that is one of the similarities it has with a genre picture.

A parallel aspect of that is the romance itself, which is far more big-R romantic, much more stylised, more melodramatic than the romances – one doesn't even use that word – than the relationships between men and women in your other films.

I think the relationship between Morgan and Jo is mainly physical. That

is not really responding to what you were saying though. . .I don't
think of it as melodramatic, it is not intended to be – you find it so?

Yes, I think so, especially beside the other films.
I did want to set up the audience's expectations that they were going
to be in for a film with heroes and heroines but then they are
frustrated because they ultimately have to evaluate these characters
themselves. The situations the *Far East* characters are facing are not
ones we normally face in Australia but they are still real. When we
were taken to meet some trade unionists in the Philippines we had to
follow 30 metres behind the person who was taking us, and while we
were talking in the back room of a restaurant everyone was incredibly
edgy that the police might suddenly burst in. In a society like that,
your relationships also probably do have something of that
heightened quality, that seen from our tranquil perspective might
seem a bit over the top. But I don't see it myself and I didn't intend it to
be melodramatic.

Was Far East *a much bigger production than you had worked on
before?*
The budget was much larger than the tiny budgets that I had worked
on before, although still only a medium-sized budget by today's
standards – it was just under $1.5 million. The crew was bigger by
about six or seven people than the crew on *Winter*.

*The clothes that the lead characters wear, particularly Peter and
Jo Reeves, are an important aspect of their larger-than-life
quality – was that something you intended?*
It is part of the subtle heightening of the reality. I had discussions
about the wardrobe with the production designer and the costume
person during the early stages and from time to time during the shoot.
But there were some costumes that weren't ready until just before
particular scenes were shot and I must admit I was quite taken aback by
a couple of them. I still have ambivalent feelings about them. One of the
costumes was the dress Helen Morse wears to the cocktail party and of
them was that pink dinner suit that Peter Reeves wears. On every other
film I have been able to see the costumes before the shoot.

You cast Bryan Brown and Helen Morse in the lead roles, who at the time were about as close as we've got in Australia to old-style movie stars, after the successs of A Town Like Alice *and all the rumours of romance between them. Was that part of the genre approach too?*

No. I think the casting was done before *A Town Like Alice* was released, though I certainly knew that they had acted in it and that they were good. In fact it was only the second thing they had done together, and innumerable people do two, three or four things together without being considered teams. There was media bombardment about them being 'reunited' that I think was a bit of overkill.

How did you cast the Filipino parts?

We wanted to try and use local actors for those roles. Richard Mason and I have never actually brought in an overseas actor, although I do think there are cases where such casting is necessary. Regarding the current controversy over union restrictions on foreign actors, I feel confident that Actors' Equity would recognise genuine cases in which the necessity for foreign cast is inherent in the script. The principal Asian role in *Far East* was Rosita. Fortunately we found Raina McKeon here in Australia and I was extremely happy with her portrayal.

How do you feel about the other Filipino parts – I'm thinking of one that struck me as less successful, the character of Bryan Brown's girlfriend, Nenay?

Yes, I think from a scripting point of view that is the weakest character in the film. The problems are in the script, not with the performer. I have done a version for overseas that has cut back fairly heavily on that character, and cut out some of the more histrionic lines I unfortunately gave her to say.

Looking back on Far East, *how successful do you think the strategy was of working in more of a genre framework than you had before? Are you as happy with the film as with others?*

It is too early for me to be entirely objective about *Far East*. I'd like to see it in a year or so. I know at the time the film was about to go out to the public, I felt very pleased with it. I was disappointed in general with the critical reaction to it – a lot of the critics attacked it and I felt that what they said often bore little relation to the film. The film did well at the box office in Australia, though not in the class of exceptional box office films like *Man from Snowy River* or *Mad Max 1* and *2*. I do take the critical reception and the reactions of people I know seriously, but in the period immediately following a film's release I think I'm not wholly rational in my response to that criticism and I did feel very angry about the way the film was received, so I can't make a particularly objective judgement about how successful it is. The film was seen by a lot of politicians in Canberra and was discussed in detail there, and I was pleased about that. When the film was shown in the San Francisco Film Festival the Filipino Consulate was ringing the agents to try and see the film for themselves and I was pleased about that because it shows they are slightly alarmed by it. I hope the film is shown to a wide audience in America because I think the debate on the human rights situation in the Philippines is limited and anything that raises the subject is useful. And I'd like to imagine that people who have seen the film and who go into a place like the Koala Klub might feel slightly differently about it. If the film makes some contribution in those areas I would feel it has been successful.

Are they the sorts of criteria by which you generally judge your films?
No, there are a great many others. I want the film to work as a piece of cinema, I want it to involve, excite and move a large audience. *Far East* seems to have polarised people, as a lot of my films do. I have had a lot of unsolicited, very positive feedback about it which makes me think that the mainstream public probably liked it a lot more than the critics did. But I was particularly irritated by a couple of Australian critics who were patronising about some of the film's images – for example the small boy staring at Morgan Keefe's boots in the penultimate scene. I remember during the Vietnam war period two mainstream audience westerns, *Little Big Man* and *Soldier Blue,* which made potent anti-war statements. Sure, there were some simple images – the cavalry galloping over a US flag on their way to slaughter the women and children of an Indian village for example – but I felt such images were totally appropriate at that time. Using

simple images doesn't involve talking down to an audience – it merely acknowledges that most people are not schooled in the intricacies of cinematic language that decorate film literature. A strong and simple image speaks to more people than the obscure symbolism that delights the esoteric critic.

R E F L E C T I N G   O N   D I R E C T I N G

W r i t i n g   t h e   P i c t u r e s

There seem to be relatively few people in Australia who both write and direct successfully – why do you think that is?
They are two quite separate areas and in this age of specialisation a lot of people come to film having learnt a particular skill in film school, or having specialised in something on television, or having worked their way up, say, from assistant directing. I always aimed to be a writer, but before I became a writer I was acting and doing some theatre directing, so the two areas were developing conjointly. I have always been interested in following through the thing that I want to write about. I am in many ways quite an obsessive writer, and the only time I am not writing is when I am actually directing a film – it is part of my life to write and has been for the last ten years.

Do you have a routine for writing?
I do have a kind of routine when my major priority is writing as opposed to pre-production, shooting, or editing. I generally work at home for a couple of hours in the morning, maybe three hours in the afternoon and maybe a couple of hours late at night. On weekday afternoons I have bets on the races, so every half hour or so I listen to a race. I find this very useful because it completely takes my mind off whatever I'm writing, and it's something I can do without spending a lot of time because I just ring up on my telephone account. I also go out for walks two or three times during the day so that breaks up the period of work. If I write for three hours solid, generally I am fairly mentally exhausted and won't feel like going back to it for the rest of the day, whereas working for 20 to 25 minutes at a time and

punctuating it with ten-minute breaks I find I can work reasonably effectively for long periods.

Do you win at the races?
Sometimes. I win and lose – it balances out roughly evenly.

How clear is the final structure when you begin writing – do you have a sense of the total duration of the film and plan, for example, that by twenty minutes so much has to have happened?
No, I don't write like that at all. Nor do I have set rules that a script has to do x, y or z for the benefit of the audience. There have been formulae produced about the minimum requirements for a successful feature film script and I have never studied them – I like to feel free to go where the ideas take me. But there are certain skills that hopefully develop, and one of them is that you get a subterranean feeling for the shape of a film and the amount of material you can carry within it. I think with *The Firm Man* for example I tried to cover far too much ground.

At what stage do you make the decision about how a particular action is to be shown?
I generally have an idea of the structure of a scene. On the actual framing and choice of lens I generally ask the camera operator. I describe what the shot is and the camera operator suggests a start-off framing, lines up the camera and says 'have a look at this, what do you think of this?' and often they have improved on my initial idea. Some of the elements are more conceptual, I would have general ideas before the shooting and develop them through rehearsal. They are usually to do with the movement of the camera or the juxtaposition of characters within an inert frame. Generally what I want to do – and most directors would think similarly – is to complement the action with the movement of the camera and some-times to use the camera to give you further information about character dynamics or the characters' relationship to a particular environment. It's a very important part of the creative machinery, because one of the key areas of decision making for the director is the way he or she actually blocks the scene, the way the characters are arranged, the way they move within the location, and the way

the camera records that. I think directors are rarely given enough credit for that by film analysts.

There are dangers in being both writer and director. You've said that you were probably a fairly self-indulgent actor, and obviously whatever dangers of indulgence there are in writing and directing are compounded by being in such a controlling position.

That is true, and you need to open yourself up to feedback from as many sources as possible. You get a lot of input from actors, your d.o.p., producer, designer, editor, sound mixer, composer, and so on – but you do have to make yourself a bit more open still because you are dealing with both jobs. I don't think there is any way of safeguarding against buggering the thing up and maybe the chances of buggering it up are slightly increased by having one person doing both jobs – but on the other hand you do get a unified vision in the directorial and script areas. What you don't get is a second person coming along taking the screenwriter's conception and complementing and adding to that – I guess you could argue that there are positives and negatives in either situation.

The   Marketplace

How important are the critics?

I think the critics do have a very significant effect on the public with certain kinds of films. The sort of film that they can have a decisive effect on is just the sort of film that I make – films which are outside the mainstream in terms of their subject matter, and are perhaps a little more demanding of an audience than a straight 'entertainment' film. They are films that are initially dependent on the 'art house' movie audience going along to see them, then they build up on word of mouth. Generally speaking they won't have enough money spent on promotion campaigns to buy an initial wave of the mainstream audience. 'Art house' audiences are those most persuaded by the critics so if you get caned by them you are in real trouble. My own personal feeling about reviews is that I do get hurt by them, I do find it difficult to completely ignore them and feel 'they just haven't understood, the fuckwits'. I think you can't help but be disappointed and sometimes made angry by critics who are tearing to shreds something that you care about a lot and have put a lot of yourself into. But it's part of the business and if you get too worried you should get out of it.

How do you feel about the way the system of distribution and exhibition works in Australia – do you think that the tie-up between distributors and exhibitors has had any effect on your films in particular and on the industry in general?
I think it has been difficult for non-mainstream films to get into the best cinemas at the best times – I think it is still difficult now. There have been certain films that have done well commercially that have helped break down that pattern – *Winter of our Dreams* and Ken Cameron's film of *Monkey Grip* are two films that are outside the mainstream but which have succeeded in getting a fair percentage of the mainstream audience. I think the most negative element about the distribution-exhibition tie up is the fact that the producer is in a weak negotiating position and gets a shockingly small amount of the ulti-mate cake. There has not really been a situation of great competition between the three major distributors for local product. The huge success of films like *Man from Snowy River* and *Mad Max* has meant that the makers of those films now have the opportunity to ask for more favourable percentages, but with the majority of films you don't really have much room for manoeuvre in what you can ask for.

Do you think the shift in film financing from the public sector to private investors will affect the possibility of making explicitly political films?
Its a bit too early to judge. Certainly when the tax concessions were first announced there was a lot of money around for films and a glut of films were made – in that atmosphere we raised the money for *Far East* very quickly. Mind you, we had some attractive incentives in our casting for both *Winter* and *Far East*: it's always easier to get investment if you have some ingredients that are well known, such as a best-selling book or actor.

The majority of the people guiding where the money goes will be attempting to make judgements on the commerciality of the material, regardless of its political content. So if you had a film extolling the

virtues of an extreme right-wing party that included the most
marvellous car chase ever, you'd probably get money for it. Likewise
if it suggested that the Russian secret police were God's gift to man
but it had the same car chase you'd probably get the money as well. I
don't think the people making judgements about whether to put tax
money into films have very different criteria from those used by the
assessors of the government film corporations. I think all of them are
trying to evaluate the commercial potential of a film, and that doesn't
get any easier. The percentage of misguided judgements is likely to be
just as high in either camp. In both cases the filmmaker has to
persuade people that there is an audience for the film.

W o r k i n g   w i t h   A c t o r s

Do you ever think about going back to acting?
Yes, I do plan to do some more acting. Probably not in films I direct
myself – I think I am a fairly self-indulgent actor and I'd need someone
outside to give me feedback on what I was doing. I would like to do
some more stage acting, really for enjoyment's sake as much as
anything – it appeals to me to act in a traditional play in an old
proscenium arch theatre for a few weeks. I love the life backstage and
the process of evolving the play and the experience of that very special
magic of working before an audience. I miss that a lot – there are
times when I'm directing actors in film when I feel a great sense of
anguish when as a director you have to move out of the circle of final
action. There is a sort of humbling moment when the pressure goes
onto the actors completely and they have to produce the goods in this
often very alienating circumstance of the film set, and there's nothing
more you as the director can do to help.

*Do you ever get that sense of connection when you are watching
one of your films with an audience?*
It is a very different though no less tangible experience, watching a film
with an audience. It is an extremely disturbing and nail-biting situation
because the film is out of your control. When you are on the stage you
can adjust your performance to an extent according to the audience's
responses, but a film has its own life at that point and all you can do is sit

there and wince or smile according to the audience's response. The first time you do sit down with an audience is a very uncomfortable experience, and I think that is probably something you never get over. Such a lot of time and effort goes into a film from a lot of people, but particularly from producers, directors, and writers. There are very few jobs where such a big span of time is finally crystallised in something that is set up for judgement by everybody else. It is fairly difficult not to feel wretched if a film you have made is not liked, because it is the summation of a long period of very hard work.

Do you rehearse for a film the same way as you do for theatre? Are any of the crew there for example?
No, just the actors. In some respects it's like theatre, but in most films you don't shoot in a continuous run like a theatre performance, so you rehearse individual scenes. It's harder in some ways because the cast is usually so much larger in a film, so you only get the chance to rehearse with the principals, and maybe you'll only have one session with people who are in for just one or two scenes.

In Winter of our Dreams *you worked with Judy Davis and Bryan Brown, who appear to be actors who approach their craft very differently – is that the case?*
Yes it is – they have very different ways of working. I'll only talk about aspects of this because I could go on at great length. One notable area is that Judy appears to remain in a similar key to a scene in the time leading up to and following the shooting of it – she gears up to the scene and takes a long time to come down from it. Bryan can be chatting away to technicians or whatever quite soon after having done a seemingly draining scene but in the moments before it he goes through quite a dramatic build-up. So when they are doing a scene there is a sense of enormous controlled pressure within both of them. Sometimes if Bryan makes a mistake, he will shout 'fuck!' The first time it happened, I thought 'good God, he is going to go into some terrible tantrum, we won't be able to shoot and I'm going to have to go away and talk him out of this for an hour or so,' but it was just like taking the lid off a pressure cooker – he immediately wants to get back into it and the control comes right back on. When Judy was playing Lou's moments of near breakdown, the distress she radiated

was palpably distressing to the crew – I can remember watching her doing those scenes and being in tears myself. The ultimate shot in the film, the long enduring close-up of her at the demonstration left a lot of the crew quite speechless.

It is the same on the screen. Did you do more than one take of that final scene?

No, just the one. I don't think we even discussed the intimate details of the final shots of each of the characters immediately before we did them. It is a cumulative thing: you do most of the detailed work in the rehearsal period and then you try to obtain what you have agreed upon in the actual shoot. But in fact we never rehearsed those final shots and I wasn't sure exactly what they were going to do in them. Of course we had talked at great length about what was going on in the heads of the characters and what was going on for them emotionally but I left it up to them to express that.

Do you usually do a number of takes of a particular scene? How unusual is it to do just one take of something like that final scene of Judy's?

We usually try especially hard to have everything completely right for shots that have difficult emotional moments in them. One of the most infuriating and taxing things for an actor is when something happens technically on one of those shots which means you have to do them again, so in general I try to keep the technical side of those moments relatively simple to try and reduce the number of things that can go wrong. As a rule we try to get all the technical problems sorted out before the actors come onto the set – that's a particular emphasis of mine as a director. Working with actors is one of the most rewarding parts of the whole filmmaking process for me, because of the central place they have in the sorts of subjects I'm interested in. If you have a film essentially about cars or armies then you will probably have just as much fun playing with the tanks and constructing the crashes.

Filmmaking and Politics

What sort of reactions have you had to Winter of our Dreams?
The film tends to polarise people. Some people find it depressing and
criticise it for not coming up with solutions. But that criticism strikes
me as simplistic to the point of idiocy. For a start the idea of a film
coming up with solutions to moral, psychological, and political
problems seems to set expectations for the media that are hopelessly
inflated. And secondly, I don't personally feel that I want to preach
through films. Providing solutions to problems like those tackled in
Winter would inevitably mean trivialising the subjects. A film is only
about one and a half to two hours long – you can't espouse a whole
philosophy containing solutions to the world's problems. It is a
medium much better suited to examining ideas and provoking trains
of thought, analysis, and evaluation.

*What sense do you have of an audience? Who do you want to
reach?*
With some of the key areas of *Winter of our Dreams* I really expected
to reach only people like the Robs and Gretels, people from that
generation, and it was particularly directed towards them. But it is
also an unrequited love story, and the contrast of the rational and
emotional ways of being-in-the-world involve anyone who goes to see
the film. So there were two quite distinct thematic elements that were
of interest to different sections of the public. I am not interested in
doing films, say, that are mainly accessible only to Marxists, as some
people accuse Godard of doing. I really am interested in reaching the
full mainstream audience.

*You've described yourself as a political filmmaker – how do you
see the political function of film?*
It is almost impossible to track down a causal connection between an
individual film and actual political change. I suppose you could
contemplate a situation where a film was exploring the implications
of a particular law that was drastically destructive to some minority
group, and the furore caused by the film put pressure on the
government and the law was changed. But generally speaking, films
operate in a much broader way as part of the social flux out of which

change comes. Films can, for example, sensitise or desensitise – I believe the preponderance of films that wallow in violence contributes to a gradually evolving insensitivity to human dignity and value. Films can reflect and therefore reinforce change – in fashions, attitudes to certain forms of behaviour or to social groups, or politics. But even a single film like *The China Syndrome,* for example, can make a major contribution to increasing the level of public awareness of an issue.

I hope my current film *One Night Stand* will be one small contribution to the anti-nuclear movement. It is more homed in on a particular issue than most of my films have been – in most of them a hell of a lot of the political component has been explored through the relationship dynamics of the principal characters and the psychological analysis involved. *One Night Stand* is a departure from that.

What sort of effect did you want Mouth to Mouth *to have?*
I wanted to depict four characters who were engaging and accessible to as large a public as possible and to suggest that they were people who had enormous potential which was not being given the opportunity to develop or flourish, and that there is a tragedy in that. It was really a quite simple intention in the case of that film – it was an attempt to bring the problem of unemployed youth up into people's consciousness. I didn't want any elements in the film that would retard people from being able to identify with the characters, no matter how different their world might be from the audience's world.

You said that you were not interested in mere entertainment – how do you understand the function of entertainment in film-making? Is it just the sugar that sweetens the pill of the message?
I think as a viewer you are unlikely to start engaging with something unless you find elements in it that are drawing you in, so it is pointless to have a film that is incredibly profound in its political analysis but which is boring. I think it is important that there is no distinction between the sugar and the medicine – that is, as a filmmaker I have to find ways of making my subjects absorbing, engaging, entertaining.

That is not merely for the pragmatic reason of it being necessary in order to get one's message across; it is saying something about the film medium and its place in society and the expectation people have of film.

You have said that you enjoy films that raise issues and make people think – who are the filmmakers that you admire?
Two would be Louis Malle and Francois Truffaut. I am impressed by the eclectic nature of Malle's subjects – he ranges over all sorts of things. My favourites among his films are *Will of the Wisp, Lacombe Lucien,* and *Murmur of the Heart.* And the thing I like most about Truffaut is the warmth of his films, the feeling that they are very frequently a celebration of quite small human beings and situations. I feel that he is a very positive filmmaker. Some of my other favourite films would be *Singing in the Rain, Casablanca, Nashville, Amarcord,* the Czech film by Jiri Menzel called *Closely Watched Trains,* the Russian science-fiction film *Solaris,* Hitchcock's *The Lady Vanishes, His Girl Friday, Midnight Cowboy, They Shoot Horses, Don't They?, A Taste of Honey* – that covers a fair bit of ground.

AN AUSTRALIAN OR MID-PACIFIC CINEMA?

Melodrama, Sexuality, and Ockerism.

The American critic Pauline Kael has accused Australian films of being dull and unchallenging – she's said that to be known as Australian in America is like having 'the Seal of Good Housekeeping'.
I think that's probably fair comment. Its probably a reflection of how in periods of recession people want to be reassured and they want uncomplicated entertainment films. That was certainly true in the thirties, the heyday of the Golddiggers films, and of the studio comedies. Perhaps in periods of economic upturn, like the sixties,

there is more likelihood of confrontation within society as a whole and a call for that to be reflected in the arts. It is a weakness in Australian films; I think there is a tendency for them to be bland. I don't think any of us as filmmakers are free from that challenge.

A lot of American critics have used words like 'fresh', 'naive' and 'innocent' to describe the Australian cinema. How accurate do you think those perceptions are?
One way in which they're accurate is that there is very little 'exploitation' in Australian films, in the sense in which that word is used in the film industry these days. You can call that naive or innocent, I suppose.

Why do you think it is that so few Australian films have had what you described as that heightened quality – there are not many characters in Australian films who have been French nightclub singers in Saigon ...
I've heard the writer Bob Ellis remark that Australia is too big for good stories, and one interpretation of that is that in some ways there is too much distance between characters for the sparks to really fly. I think if scripts exhibit this it is because the writers are reflecting an Australian tendency to draw back from confrontational emotional situations. I don't think this is because the situations are absent from our history and our contemporary culture, I think it's that we are a bit reluctant to confront them or depict them with their full force.

Why do you think that is?
I think it is maybe because we don't like to show emotion, we don't like to cry publicly. It is to do with our masculine-derived cultural identity as Australians – that it is effeminate to show vulnerabilities or even to talk in detail about a painful situation that we might be encountering. And probably because we find it difficult to talk about, it is harder for filmmakers to show it – maybe we are collectively reflecting the shortcomings of our national identity.

Your films are fairly unusual in that they do directly address emotional questions and questions to do with sexuality – why do you think that's so rare in Australian filmmaking?

Perhaps it reflects the way the subject of sex is traditionally treated in Australia, at a bawdy surface level, with talks of male prowess in pubs, so you get the trivialisation of sexuality in films like *Alvin Purple* and by television characters like Paul Hogan. The way in which sexuality appears in those situations is not really related to actual sexuality at all – it is a trivialised version of it. Combined with the fact that there isn't any comparable mature depiction or discussion of sexual matters, I think that suggests that there is a reticence and unease about sexuality. That's not particularly unusual in Western countries recovering from the Victorian era, but maybe it's more pronounced in Australia because of our history – we began as a society in which women were at a premium, which perhaps started off the mateship ethos. It meant that men had to deal largely or solely with other men, and to deal with a woman was exceptional, so sexuality gained a heightened or unreal quality which in turn gives rise to stories that get encapsulated into bar-room myth and are celebrated in poem, song, and subsequently television and film. I think that pattern is being gradually eroded but I think it is still exerting a significant influence.

There are very few macho heroes of the classic mould in Australian films which is paradoxical in a way.
Yes, some years ago Phillip Adams came up with the idea that the male characters in Australian films were dominated by reticent men. I think there is some truth in that: maybe it is an artist's response to the identity I was alluding to before. Rather than reproduce that crass, demeaned view of sexuality in the characters we may have tended to concentrate on the feelings of anxiety or inadequacy that underlie it – and that could make them appear sheepish.

I'm not sure that the reason that we have such reticent male heroes in the films is simply to do with the delicacy of the filmmakers in not wanting to show the bravado and so on.
We are generalising of course – there are films that are notable exceptions to all this. But when you think of the first wave of films that were made, apart from the odd exceptions like *Picnic at Hanging Rock* and *Caddie*, they were very frequently dominated by the ocker identity – look at *Alvin Purple, Alvin Rides Again, Don's*

*Party, Barry McKenzie, Barry McKenzie Holds His Own,
Petersen, Sunday Too Far Away* ... it becomes hard to find films
whose male characters are *not* roughly in that area. And there was
really a very strong critical outcry which as I said hit *Dimboola* – the
critics wanted to see Australians depicted as sensitive, mature,
educated people. So that may be another reason, maybe
unconsciously, for some filmmakers drawing back from depicting too
many Australians in their full crass truth. I'm not saying that
Australians are in the main gross ockers but the ocker aspect of
Australians is nevertheless extraordinarily common, and it reappears
persistently in Australian society and in Australian mainstream
television.

Do you see any of that in the two boys in Mouth to Mouth?
There are flashes in it. I think that what happens when ockers are
depicted on television and film in general is that their most gross
surface features are dwelt upon to the exclusion of all else. In fact the
ocker is no less complex a personality than any other, and has dreams
and fears and passions and paranoias the same as the sharply dressed
Frenchman who chases girls around Paris in French films. In the
early films those other dimensions of that character were not really
dwelt upon as much as they might have been, though there were
glimpses in some of the characters in *Don's Party* and *Petersen*. But
the picture that was being furthered by the critics was that ockers
were just gross oafs and bore very little relationship at all to the reality
of Australian society, and that is just simply inaccurate on both
counts.

*I wonder if one of the reasons Bryan Brown was so enthusias-
tically embraced as an actor coming just after that period is that
he captures a lot of those quintessentially Australian male
characteristics without many of the unpleasant aspects.*
Yes, I think that is part of why he is so popular. Though I think a large
number of the 'art house' audience would still prefer to see
themselves mirrored on the screen by a Trintignant type ... but I
think they should probably go and live in France.

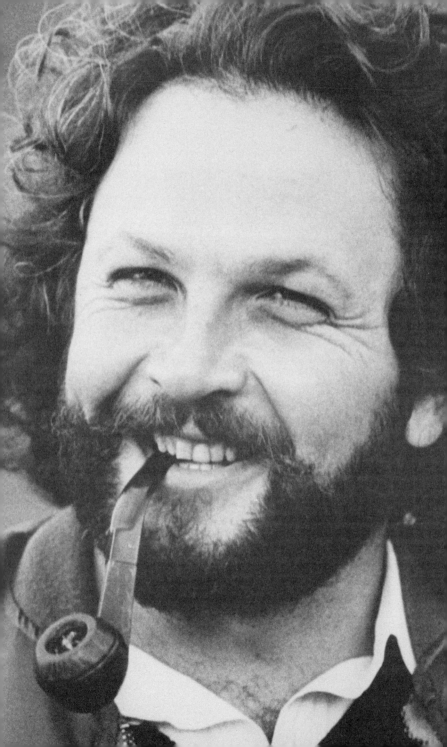

GEORGE MILLER

George Miller's genial and gentle demeanour confounds expectations that the director of the most taut and violent films made in Australia would have a personality to match. He is a loquacious talker and you get the impression that he is often thinking two or three steps ahead of his words as they form themselves into long, sometimes rambling sentences. Having begun an answer he will often digress with examples, side issues, and other people's insights before coming back to the original question. A plumpish man with unmodishly long hair, he admits ruefully to a passion for chocolates.

This interview took place in three different locations. The first was in Sydney, in a small video-editing room where Miller was absorbed in cutting his episode of *The Dismissal,* the six-part television series made in 1982 about the 1975 sacking of the Australian Labor government. Miller had been up most of the night before, but it was only later, listening to the tape play back, that the exhaustion in his voice became evident. His conversation was friendly, lucid, and spilling over with ideas.

The second instalment took place some six months later, when Miller was in Hollywood directing a segment of Stephen Spielberg's *The Twilight Zone.* 'I think he's going to wrap today,' a secretary versed in film jargon had told me, and indeed when I spoke to Miller shooting had just been completed. He was in a mildly euphoric state, full of enthusiasm for the film's crew, who had willingly agreed to come back on a Sunday to reshoot a crucial scene. After meeting in the *Twilight Zone* office at the Warner Brothers studio lot, most of the interview took place in a Burbank restaurant. Miller expressed surprise at the degree to which his prejudices about Hollywood had been challenged by actually working there. 'I realised there are about ten Hollywoods,' he said, 'and you can choose the one you want to play in. In fact, you can almost pick them by the restaurants they eat at.' I didn't ask about the significance of the straightforward cafe he'd

225

chosen, but its lace tablecloths located it somewhere between the paper mats of the regular diner and the salmon-pink linen of the fashionably expensive Hollywood eating spots.

The third conversation took place at Miller's home base, the Metro Theatre in Sydney's Kings Cross, next door to the offices of Actors' Equity. The Metro Theatre is the headquarters of Kennedy Miller Pty Ltd, the production company formed by Miller and producer Byron Kennedy, who was killed in a helicopter accident in July 1983. Since its formation the organisation has expanded to include the writer Terry Hayes, whose collaboration with Miller began when he was assigned to write the 'novelisation' of *Mad Max,* the very successful 1979 film that was Miller and Kennedy's first feature. Hayes and Miller together wrote the screenplay for the sequel, *Mad Max 2* (1981), which has become the most successful Australian film to date in the US where it was distributed by Warner Brothers under the title *The Road Warrior. Mad Max 2* continued the explosive montage-based style that had made *Mad Max* an immediate classic of the car-action genre. For some time considered not quite 'proper' candidates to join the ranks of the most respected Australian films, the enormous popularity of both *Mad Max* and *Mad Max 2* eventually overcame the delicate sensibilities of Australia's critical establishment.

Kennedy Miller 'has sort of slowly grown,' says Miller. 'At first it was just Byron and I, then Terry came in and now there's George Ogilvie as well.' At the time of the interview Ogilvie, a well-known theatre director and former lecturer at the National Institute for Dramatic Art, was supervising a series of workshops attended by actors, writers and directors (Gillian Armstrong was one of those in attendance). The workshops were being organised 'to no other end than just to enquire, to try and shed light on some questions we want answered,' explained Miller. 'For instance, why do we so rarely achieve the sense you get in some movies made in New York, for example, that everyone is acting in the same picture, that everyone seems to be on the same train. And why it is some performances ring true, they resonate and you can believe them, while others you just can't.'

Kennedy Miller has seen itself not simply as a private entrepreneurial organisation, but as part of a film community, and the impact of Byron Kennedy's tragic death at 32 was felt throughout the film industry. This interview had been concluded not long before and it is obvious that Kennedy's death meant the end of what had been an extraordinarily creative partnership.

In Australia, where most directors work as independent operators, moving from project to project, the Kennedy Miller organisation has been unique. The organisation provides Miller with a buffer against the vagaries of freelance work, and its integrated operation affords him greater involvement in the entire process of filmmaking than is available to most freelance directors. On the door of Miller's office is a sign inscribed 'Manager', a leftover from the days when the Metro actually functioned as a cinema. The walls are bare. At one end of the room is a washbasin which creates an impression oddly reminiscent of a doctor's surgery; at the other end are bookshelves containing volumes of science fiction and horror stories, film texts, art book and Hitchcock screenplays. One shelf contains an eclectic assortment of contemporary works ranging from *Zen and the Art of Motorcycle Maintenance* through *Kinflicks* and *Nympho and Other Maniacs* to older classics like *Three Men in a Boat* and *The Grapes of Wrath*. There's a volume of Leunig cartoons, Bill Wannon's *The Australians,* and on the top shelf are seven copies of Joseph Campbell's *The Masks of God: Primitive Mythology.*

There is very little of the egocentric 'star director' about Miller. He has a highly rationalised perspective on filmmaking that provides a way of approaching everything from the most broadly philosophical issues to the most immediate technical and financial practicalities. He will argue his view tenaciously but without the rancour of insecurity, and he has a curiosity and interest in things around him that are rare in the film world. Though he maintains that he usually avoids interviews, Miller was remarkably generous with his time. The chance to talk at length and to share information about the craft of filmmaking seemed, he explained, a worthwhile exercise. In approving the edited transcript, Miller made only minor corrections and clarifications, and expanded the account of the *Mad Max* hospital sequence he had used to explain his concept of story. He requested the deletion of some details about his childhood, on the ground that people make assumptions on the basis of things they read which can interfere with the development of good working relationships. Even his attitude to personal revelation comes down to what he calls his bottom line – 'it all rests in the work.'

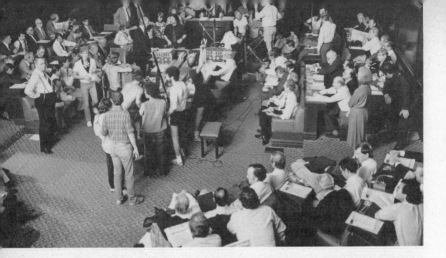

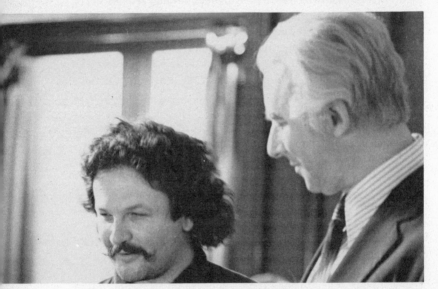

Above: Cast and crew in place on the Parliament House set of *The Dismissal*. George Miller is standing in front and just to the right of the Speaker's table.

Below: 'In general I've been one of those people who likes to think of themselves as staying outside the political process and observing it . . . and yet somehow of course we *are* all involved.' George Miller and Max Phipps as Prime Minister Gough Whitlam on the set of *The Dismissal*.

Right: 'We used the car chases as the ritual of death, rather than the guns and shootouts of the westerns or the swordfights of the Samurai films.' George Miller, Mel Gibson and car.

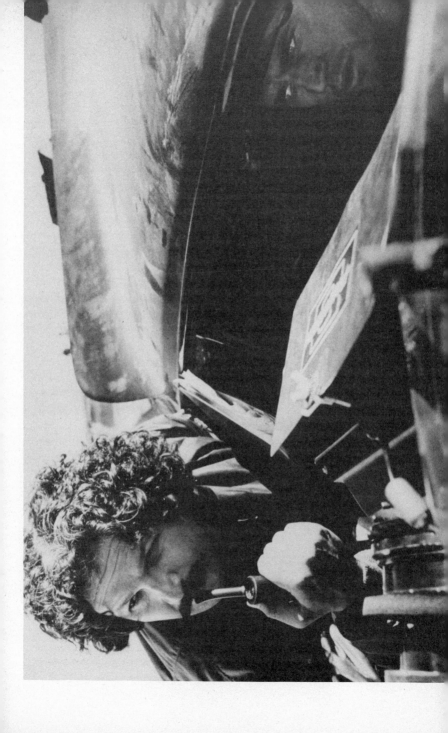

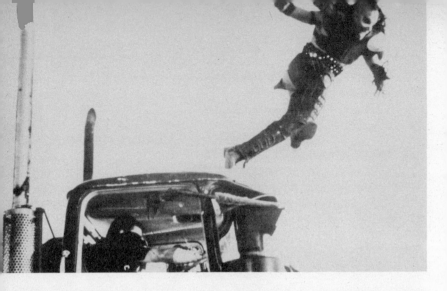

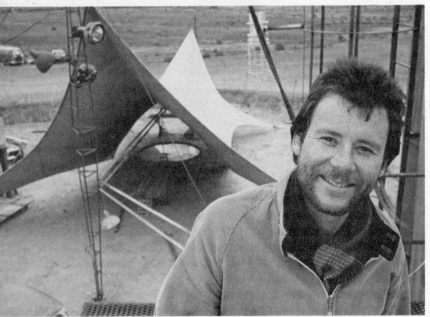

Above: 'You can have so much more fun with the bad guys.'
Vern Wells as Wez in *Mad Max 2 (The Road Warrior).*

Below: Byron Kennedy on the set of *Mad Max 2.*

BEGINNINGS

A Passion for Pictures

Sue Mathews: Why do you think it is that Australia has managed to produce so many successful films in the last decade?
George Miller: One of the key reasons, and the big attraction of working in Australia, has been that not much gets in the way of the filmmaking. The biggest problem in the traditional American film industry, apart from the huge costs, is the enormous machine, where everything conspires to get in the way of the film. We've all heard stories of how a screenplay will be modified to attract a star, or something has to be changed to fit what the market research says audiences want that week, and the original vision or purpose gets distorted in the process. It will happen in Australia, but because we're such an immature industry it happens much less.

So if someone has a very strong, passionate need to make a particular film, to tell a particular story, they are much more likely to be able to get it done and have it come out the other end with the passion intact. I'm not talking about the actual content of the film, I'm talking about the passion of the filmmaker – whether a producer, director, writer, whoever is the principal driving force behind the film – to make a particular film. *My Brilliant Career* is a fine example: the producer, Margaret Fink, and I presume the director, Gillian Armstrong as well, were hawking that film around for ages, reworking draft after draft, until finally the only thing they had left was an absolute need to make that film. It was the same with *Gallipoli* which I admire a lot. Peter Weir was absolutely determined that he was going to make that film, and it took five years, but he eventually got to make the film he wanted to make. That's the kind of passion I'm talking about.

Why does someone get passionate about a film like Mad Max?
There was a big difference between the origins of the two *Mad Max* films. With the first *Mad Max* the passion was making a low-budget genre film involving action, a Roger Corman-type B-grade movie, and doing it the best we could. It might be 'exploitation' filmmaking but I

can tell you that the producer, Byron Kennedy, and I absolutely sweated blood on that film for a long time. The first thing is that you get addicted to the filmmaking process. People who were making films in Australia in the early days were making films because they had to, not because it was a good career – it didn't even exist as a career. Phil Noyce, for example, was waving Bolexes around back at school and would do anything to work on a film in some capacity, he was just addicted to the process, and I think that was the thing for most of us. You couldn't make a living from it, except if you made commercials or worked for Film Australia or the ABC, but there was this need to make films. Maybe 'passion' is not the right word, maybe it is obsession, addiction. It was so difficult to make a film early on here, you had to take so many 'nos' from people that it really tested out whether or not you wanted that story to be made. On *Mad Max* it took a year and hundreds of 'nos' just on financing. And of course Byron and I had never made a film before – I had never even been on a movie set before.

What had you been doing up till then?
I came to the film industry pretty late. I was a medical graduate, and I was working as a resident in a hospital. I had been a film buff all my life but I never imagined that I would ever get practically involved in the film industry. I spent most of my six years at medical school at the movies – I have a twin brother who went to medical school with me and he was a much faster and neater writer than I was, so he was able to take all the notes which meant I was at nearly every eleven o'clock session of the movies for six years. Then in 1970 there was a film competition at NSW University – you had one hour in one room to make a one-minute, black-and-white film. One of my younger brothers entered the competition with a little film we had devised and it happened to win. The prize was to go to a film workshop at Melbourne University, and since that summer I was waiting around to commence residency in a hospital, I thought 'if he's going I should go too'.

That was where I met Byron Kennedy and we've been making films ever since. Phil Noyce was the person who taught me to use a camera at that workshop. I worked for two years in a hospital but whenever I had a break we'd go off and make a little experimental film somewhere, or record sound on someone's film, or cut someone's documentary, anything. In 1971 Byron and I made an experimental short, a little satire called *Violence in the Cinema Part 1*. It was shown at the Sydney Film Festival and as a result Greater Union asked if they could distribute the film – I didn't even know what distribution meant, I honestly didn't. We decided then to sit down and really find out what the movie business was about, and we did – but it took us until 1976 to make our first film. We earned about $92 between us in six years.

Do you think you brought anything useful from your medical training to your filmmaking?

Probably the best thing about having done medicine was that it kept me away from film for so long. I had time to see the world differently, I was more mature than if I had gone into the film industry early. Also in medicine you tend to see people in fairly extreme states and that is pretty provocative for any individual. It forces you to grapple with things you might not otherwise have to confront.

Storytelling

After you had made Mad Max *you spent some time living in America – what drew you there?*

Terry Hayes, the writer, and I were there to oversee the release of *Mad Max* and we realised that the global film industry germinates in Los Angeles. There was so much we needed to know and it seemed the ideal place to learn – people there were so open, you could go to whoever you wanted to get information, you could find whatever books you wanted, you could see whatever movie you wanted. If you wanted the original screenplay of a Hitchcock movie you could find it somewhere: you could see that Alfred Hitchcock had scenes in mind that were in the shooting script but were never on the screen. I even did a short acting course at UCLA because I wanted to understand more about acting. But the main thing was that Terry and I found out about Joseph Campbell, who had studied comparative religion and at one stage was Jung's editor.

Campbell wrote a book called *Hero with a Thousand Faces* and in that he distilled all the hero mythologies into one model – it was on that George Lucas modelled the *Star Wars* stories. Campbell saw the function of storytellers as very basic, saying that stories are shared by different cultures throughout all time and space, and that through that process we are given access to the totality of human experience. You and I as individuals are not likely to share all the experiences available to humankind but somehow myths distill experience and put us in touch with what is eternal in man. So stories are told spontaneously over and over again – if we suddenly ended up in caves again we'd sit around telling the same stories to each other around fires. George Lucas won't be remembered as a filmmaker, he'll be remembered as the mythmaker or storyteller of this generation; instead of sitting around the fire he is using the high technology of film.

You see, *Mad Max* had succeeded in a strange mixture of cultures, from Mexico to Switzerland to Australia. It just didn't make any sense so we started to ask why. Initially people would say 'oh well, it's a violent film, it's got a lot of action, people can understand car crashes in almost every language.' But it is a bit more than that: when we went to Japan people would start talking about Samurais, in Italy they would start referring to spaghetti Westerns, in Scandinavia – Viking folklore. Of course, all these stories are really the same stories, and we realised that unconsciously we had struck a lot of mythological chords. The way these stories arise out of the filmmaker is not a conscious thing, that is the scary thing about it – those of us who did *Mad Max 1* were the unwitting servants of the collective unconscious, we definitely were, and for someone who was fairly mechanistic in his approach to life, for whom everything conformed to the laws of physics and chemistry, it is quite confronting for me to be suddenly made aware of the workings of mythology and I'm in wonder of it.

Growing   Up   with   Pop   Culture

People have commented on the way the Mad Max *films connect with other forms of popular culture, and I read about a film you were working on about pop music, called* Roxanne. *How interested are you in rock music? What was the* Roxanne *project?*

Roxanne is a screenplay Terry Hayes and I have written, and rock and roll is one of the major elements in it. I don't think you can have grown up in the fifties and sixties and not have rock and roll as one of the major parts of your life, so of course I am interested in it. The biggest influences on me have always been the pop cultures, I have never been highbrow. When I was interested in art, I leant towards the pop arts, comic books and graphics rather than high art. It has become much more blurred since the fifties and sixties – it was not too long ago that you would have a classical composer refusing to have anything to do with electronic music or jazz or even rock and roll, but look at how they are mixed up together now, and how much richer everyone is for it. As a filmmaker you are working in the popular field – filmmakers are much more vulgarian than they are high art. It's interesting to think about theatre: it was at its richest and most effective when it was made by vagabonds and whores, that crude popular theatre. When it was elevated into high art, when it got a bit toney, it lost much of its effectiveness. Theatre really has very little to do with mainstream Australian life today – and tragically I think that is happening to film, I think film has become a little bit too toney.

Did you have a strong interest in pop culture as a kid?
Well, I grew up in the country, in Chinchilla in western Queensland. In the fifties the only technology we had that gave us access to those things was radio, newspapers, and cinema – the only thing we knew of America was from the Saturday matinees. There was no television in the country at that stage, and every Saturday afternoon we'd go to the pictures, with just about every other kid in town, and see the cartoon, the serial, the B feature and the A feature. For the rest of the week, if you didn't listen to the serials on the radio, you'd go outside and act out what you'd seen at the pictures. If there was a Sir Galahad serial we'd all be running around with garbage bin lids and horses with sheets on them painted up, having jousting competitions. I was also a great reader of comics … I had a very rich fantasy childhood. There was a sense of connection with mainstream Australian culture though – we'd listen to Jack Davey on the radio, and eat Vegemite.

Did your parents try to discourage you from those pursuits?
Parents and teachers always seemed to think there was something inherently evil about comic books, that if you got addicted to comic

books – and I was, I always had a comic book slotted inside the exercise books – there was something wrong with you. I'm not very literate at all: I am an incredibly slow reader, and I have difficulty organising words, so I was visually adept rather than verbally adept, which I always took as a sign of mental inferiority.

MAKING THE MOVIES

Mad Max

What decided you to try to make an action genre picture like Mad Max?

Well, after *Violence in the Cinema* we realised that in the real world there was no place for short films, except as a way of honing your skills, and that if you wanted to make movies you had to make something of feature length. Byron had grown up in the western suburbs of Melbourne and was very interested in cars and the culture of cars and I had some of that from growing up in a country town. Working in the hospital I had developed a morbid fascination with the autocide we practise in our society: every weekend I'd see so many young people who'd been killed, or maimed for life, on the roads. You'd see the road toll in the paper on Monday morning and it was accepted with a shrug. It was almost like a weekly ritual, with people being randomly selected out as victims, as sacrifices to the car and the road.

But the film seems to be a celebration of those things – the excitement of speed and the intensity of the experience of the road.

Maybe that's the form getting in the way of the content. I can't stand slow films – in fact I think *Mad Max* is too slow. For me chases are one of the purest forms of cinema, because they only exist on film, they never exist in reality. There were never any car chases in *Mad Max*, we didn't stage a chase at Broken Hill: they were little pieces of film put together in a movie theatre. As a craft exercise it is a wonderful thing to attempt because it gives you an understanding of what film is about. We have forgotten that kinetic quality of film, how the rhythm of those bits of film creates what you can almost call visual music.

Are you saying that Mad Max *was intended as a critique of the road toll?*
No. The bizarre ritual of the road toll was the kickoff – the germinating idea as it were. Our preoccupation with chase movies was another key. The film evolved slowly out of these two impulses. We set it in the future, exaggerated it. It allowed us to tell a very simple story, like a Western. We used the car chases as the ritual of death, rather than the guns and shoot-outs of the westerns, or the swordfights in the Samurai movies. I think the sociological content comes, like most themes in a film, in a fairly unconscious way. The storyteller's attitude to the subject does seep through. I don't believe it is consciously imposed. At least it wasn't with *Mad Max I.*

To tell you the truth, I never really knew what *Mad Max* was about, at its core, until long after it was finished. It came more out of the intuition than the intellect. I've learnt now that isn't the way one should go about it. The intuition, your gut instincts, attract you to the story. The intellect strives to understand it at its core; the intellect dismantles the story to its elements, prepares it and then the intuition takes over again and shoots the movie for you.

Mad Max *is basically a revenge story – what makes you passionate about a story like that?*
The driving impulses in *Mad Max I* came out of the road toll and wanting to do a car-action picture the very best we could. The revenge story somehow generated out of that. The movie tells of people in extreme states. People who live in a Darwinian, survival-of-the-fittest world – the rules are simple and the people work on a much more primitive level than they would in a more naturalistic, contemporary drama. *Mad Max* is a metaphor – a film story – about the dark side of ourselves.

What are your interests in making genre films like Mad Max *and* Mad Max 2? *How do you want people to walk out of the theatre?*
First of all I want them to feel that they have been through an experience like being on a roller-coaster ride. I feel a sense of a job well

done when people walk out exhausted at the end. I feel good when I walk out exhausted from a movie, when I've been completely turned around or absorbed entirely, sucked into the screen. *Mad Max* and *Mad Max 2* had very different motivations. *Mad Max* was a bitter experience, it was so tough to make: it felt like I was taking a big dog for a walk, I wanted it to go in one direction and it dragged me off in another. I thought 'God, filmmaking is so hard'. I had pre-visualised the film very strongly and the film I had in my head was nothing to do with the film that was eventually on the screen, so I had a great sense of failure on that film.

What were the gaps between your vision and the final product?
The gaps were enormous – I can't begin to list them. I honestly can't even see the film any more because it was so tough. Six days into our shoot the original leading lady and our stunt co-ordinator were driving to the set at six o'clock in the morning and hit a truck. Both broke legs which meant that she was out of the film, though luckily the stunt co-ordinator Grant Page was back on the film within three weeks. Joanne Samuel, the new actress, was doing a soap opera and the producer very kindly wrote her out of the plot, but it took two weeks which completely threw our schedule out. On a low budget, that was absolutely critical so I had to make what I thought were terrible compromises. For a long time while we were cutting it I thought the film was not releasable. Byron and I virtually edited it in our lounge room because we ran out of time and money to be able to pay the editors, and Byron cut all the soundtrack himself. But then to my great surprise the film turned around and did remarkably well – it succeeded in every territory but the United States.

How did you raise the money?
We knew that we were going to have difficulty raising money, partly because we didn't have a track record, and partly because the kinds of things we wanted to make were in that 'exploitation' area that no government body would feel comfortable investing in. So we went to Graham Burke, the manager of Roadshow, one of the three major distribution companies, because we knew we had to get distributor involvement up front. Graham is one of the unsung heroes of the Australian film industry and he was very wise and realised that we had

a lot of bright talk but not much substance behind us so he said 'if you can convince some other people to invest in the film, I will match that and get involved.'

Byron drew up a presentation which was very soundly based on commerce. My tendency was to hype it and come on with all the bullshit about how wonderful film is, but Byron saw that the approach had to be on a strong commercial basis, understanding that film is always risk capital and that you can't present it as anything other than that. When people get involved they should know they are taking a punt. We went to friends and friends of friends, and the money came mostly in small lots. For instance, the secretary who typed the screenplay, invested with her sister and her husband, in lots of $2500. The biggest investment was around $15 000.

How were you supporting yourselves?
I was doing locums. We had an old van and Byron would be on the radio taking the calls and driving me from one house to another. It is the worst kind of medicine because you never get to see the patient again. But the great thing about those days was that because you had to do everything, you got a very general, comprehensive approach to making films.

Was Terry Hayes involved in writing Mad Max?
No – we met Terry when he was commissioned to write the novelisation of *Mad Max*. James McCauseland wrote the screenplay with me – he was a journalist working for *The Australian*, but now he is lost to screen writing because he has become an editor of *The Age*. It's a pity – I have a theory that journalists make the best screenwriters.

Doing a film with so many stunts in it seems a very risky thing to attempt for a first film when you had never even been on a set before. There is a picture in Cinema Papers *of you leaning off the back of a moving truck directing the cameraman ...*
I wasn't the person who had to *do* the stunts. Grant Page, the stunt co-ordinator, and most of the people working with him were very experienced – a lot of that work had been done before in Australian films or TV programs. The big problem was doing it for the budget – it

was a continual battle to repair the cars and get them going just enough to gather speed to do the stunt. Byron and I had studied stunt and chase movies – we would put them up on editing benches and go through them and see that the cars didn't really do all that, it was done through cuts and speeding up this bit of film and slowing down that and intercutting a screaming face that had been shot in a studio. So it wasn't the repertoire of stunts of *Mad Max* that was much more complex or difficult, it was devising the way they should go together. In my daily life or habits I'm not much of a risk taker – I don't go up in Byron's helicopter very often, because I know there is a certain danger in helicopters. But when the film is on I find I am there in the thick of it – there is this strange sensation when you are looking through the lens, you feel somehow insulated from the danger.

Were many of the ideas in the film things you had had in your mind for a long time, just waiting to be put in a movie?
You often have ideas for stunts, or scenes – moments in your mind, from previous projects or from anywhere at all. So there were some things that were conceived long before we had even thought of *Mad Max*, but they were used only if they answered the problem in a particular moment of the story.

One very effective stunt is when the Toecutter, the bikie leader, meets his fate – he collides with a semi-trailer and from a distance the camera watches the truck bumping over him. How was that developed?
The story requires that the Toecutter finally be destroyed, so you ask 'what would be a really terrible thing for him?' There is an old bit of bikie folklore, an apocryphal story about a bikie going between what he thinks are two other bikes' headlights, but are actually the lights of a truck, and that seemed appropriately horrendous and final.

We didn't have the scene at night, but we drew on that idea of someone hitting a truck. First you work out if it is possible to do it – there would be a huge impact for instance, but you can't really do that with stuntmen. So you devise little bits of film instead – that stunt works not just because of the actual stunt but because of the seven or eight little bits of film that precede it. They include a special effect of prosthetic eyes on a dummy that was shot in our lounge room; a shot of Byron Kennedy and his mother driving in the background in a black car; and in post-production we did a shot with a scratch crew, of Bryron with a helmet on, being held on the back of a trailer with the front piece of a motorbike in front of him, pulling off his goggles. That is just four or five frames combined with shots we did during the main body of the shoot, and a speeded-up shot of an approaching truck. The final stunt was a lot due to serendipity – it was the cheapest stunt we did and it involved work done by Steve Amezdroz and Jon Dowding, who built the dummy motorbike for the truck to hit. The dummy happened to be made of chicken wire and some other junk and the way it fell seemed very realistic – if it hadn't fallen that way we would have cut out sooner. So that whole sequence was a combination of complex things. If there was not an emotional investment in the characters it wouldn't work either, that's another aspect. It is only in the context of other little bits of film that stunts work. We had to devise it through montage. That's the great attraction for me of the silent films: look at the things Harold Lloyd and Buster Keaton did through montage.

Another grisly moment is when Johnny Boy is killed: Max puts him in a ghastly no-win situation where he has to cut off his own foot if he is to escape being burnt to death – was that something you had seen in a film before?
We thought, well, Max has changed from a relatively normal man into a monster, so he must *be* monstrous. There is the mechanical mayhem he commits earlier on, but there has to be that psychological violence, which is probably darker. I think that idea came from an old sexually-oriented joke I had heard and I thought that was a pretty horrible thing. Actually a lot of people argued that the ending should have been reversed, that the Toecutter stunt should have come last, because it turned out to be so spectacular. So you really do draw from everywhere.

The bikie gang are very theatrical, very stylised in their accents and the way they deliver their lines – they're almost melodrama villains. What was the intention there?
We tried to play with language, with accents and rhythms, a little bit more than ended up in the film – we were keying off *Clockwork*

Orange but were nowhere near as successful as that. We didn't rehearse in *Mad Max,* so it came basically from the actors. Hugh Keays-Byrne swaps accents deliberately, as part of the Toecutter's craziness – how he talked depended on how he felt, so no one could pin him down. Sometimes he spoke with a southern American accent, then an almost Shakespearean style, then in a lot of different ways. It was a way of suggesting the chaos of people losing any roots. Through all the cutting, most of which I remember very negatively, the way Hugh spoke was one of the few joys, and his delivery of a few lines rings in my ears now, after all this time.

The other thing that is theatrical about the gang is all their tumbling and acrobatics.
That is something the actors contributed. There were guys like David Bracks who had been a stunt man and was very physical. And they were all very fine bike riders.

Those theatrical elements ought to be distancing for the audience but in fact they add to how disturbing we find it.
It comes from the nature of the characters. A great deal of that is Hugh Keays-Byrne: he insisted on the bikes being sent up to Sydney (we were filming in Melbourne), and they all rode down together before the shoot, in their costumes and camping out – by the time they arrived in Melbourne they *were* the Toecutter gang. One of the reasons for that theatricality – and it is brought more into relief in *Mad Max 2* – is that when you are living in that very primitive world as a warrior, the kind that chooses to rampantly take and consume, it is much more efficient to be flamboyant and dramatic because you don't have to spend so much energy physically fighting. It is like the pageantry of all warring people, from the Nazis to a New Guinea tribe fighting a ritual war.

The other thing about the gang is their sexual ambivalence – why is that so strong?
I can remember much more clearly how it came out in *Mad Max 2* – both films have the same kind of gangs. We wanted to avoid the cliché of the modern day bikie gang that you saw in Roger Corman movies of the sixties, with the biker and his old lady. To have homosexuality amongst some of the members of the gang played off that cliché.

It also plays off against the wholesomeness of Max's family. The wife and child actually have a much bigger role in Mad Max *than in a lot of American films in that genre.*

I'm afraid I've blanked a lot of *Mad Max* out – I can't remember a lot of the decisions we made there. It's a story of a relatively normal man in a society in which the normal conventions are beginning to break down. And no matter how he tries to escape the barbarism, and preserve a wife and family, once the decay has begun even those things can't survive. A lot of it is such basic stuff – *Mad Max* is to do with much deeper, darker things than a naturalistic commentary on everyday life. Things like the bonding between mother and child and father, and questions of living and dying, are very primitive, and they are basic to much more primitive forms of storytelling. I guess it works because if it's done reasonably well it always works – there's an almost physiological response to those things.

Mad Max 2

Why did you decide to make Mad Max 2 – *were you equally passionate about that?*

We had been very unwilling to get involved with a *Mad Max 2* – there was a lot of financial pressure, and distributors from all over the world were saying 'make another one'. But it is so hard to make a film, to energise yourself and once you are doing it for money rather than because you need to make the film you are really in trouble – you can end up with very cynical sequels. But *Mad Max* had been so unsatisfactory from my point of view, and *Mad Max 2* was a chance to do the film again and perhaps do it properly because we had a much bigger budget and much more experience. This time we wanted to make it more consciously mythological – more focused. We were grappling in the dark a little less, that is what energised *Mad Max 2*.

Between Mad Max *and* Mad Max 2 *the scale of the production changed enormously – what were the differences for you in the actual making of the film?*

I think the budget was almost nine times larger in the second film.

There were several reasons for that: first, budgets over that four-year period tripled in Australia; second, in *Mad Max* we did everything on the cheap, to the point where if a script had to be delivered either Byron Kennedy or myself delivered it in a little van instead of getting a courier. For me as a director the larger budget meant that we could seek out any location we wanted in Australia. We were able to shoot it in the winter – in most of Australia it would have rained too much for a film that is almost exclusively outdoors but we were able to go to a place where the rainfall was relatively low and take the whole crew. *Mad Max* had been shot within 30 kilometres of Melbourne – we would commute there each day and we would have to carefully select our angles so you couldn't see a factory or a house, or powerlines in the background; in Broken Hill where we made *Mad Max 2* we didn't have to do that. The other big difference was that the crew was much bigger. And in post-production we had a total of five editors – at one stage we were using four editing rooms, running from one to the other, whereas *Mad Max* we virtually had to cut ourselves.

Was writing the second screenplay a very different experience from writing the first one?
Yes it was. *Mad Max 2* came out of a period when Terry Hayes and I were working on the *Roxanne* screenplay. Almost to avoid work on *Roxanne* we would start talking about the *Mad Max* story and what the character could have become. So a story started to evolve almost indirectly whereas in *Mad Max 1* the car chase narrative was the first thing we had. A lot of people said there was no screenplay involved in *Mad Max 2* because there was so little dialogue – the Max character speaks only about twenty lines altogether – but in fact a lot of work went into the screenplay, working out the core around which we dressed the rest of the picture. Terry came to the location with us to see what it was like which was very lucky because we were writing and changing the screenplay right up to the end. In fact we ran out of screenplay about the second last week of the shooting – we knew what the ending would be, but not exactly how we were going to get there, so one day we did a Francis Ford Coppola and sent the crew off to shoot shots of wheels and things while Terry and I were pounding away in the caravan trying to figure out what would happen next.

You were shooting in sequence?

Yes, which is a wonderful way to work. It was not any more expensive to shoot in sequence, and because it was a fairly linear story in which vehicles and other things were being destroyed gradually, you were actually obliged to shoot in a kind of sequence. It is a big help.

Why did you decide not to have Max join the convoy to the better life in the north in Mad Max 2?

The decision was made unconsciously: for some reason your intuition tells you that it would be terrible for him if he went with them. If you look at it a little more you will see that the hero of mythology is often, though not always, the reluctant servant of a greater purpose. Max himself is lost – he is completely burnt out at the beginning and goes through the whole film like that. There might be a spark of rehumanisation, but he has decided not to be a human being at all and he resents anything about him that is human because it has caused him so much pain in the past. Max did not belong with those people, and they themselves are really serving a purpose beyond their own survival, the establishment of a new order, rejuvenation. In all those stories, from the outlaw samurai who always continues to wander, to the gunslinger riding off into the sunset time and time again, there is a feeling of rightness about that conclusion, and to go against that just didn't seem right.

You take the homosexual dimensions of the bikie gang a lot further in Mad Max 2 than in the first film.

Yes. Now that we've done that twice I have to admit there might be an unconscious response there. In *Mad Max 2,* the plot demanded someone on the back of the Wes character's bike, who would be killed by the little boy. We had written it as a woman but it just didn't seem right, it brought us back to those sixties movies every time, so we made the character a boy. The s & m gear was designed by Norma Moriceau who lived next door to, and was influenced by, the Link, an s & m leather shop in Sydney. There were quite a few women in the gang but we decided there should not be any sexual differentiation, so most of the women were wearing leather and helmets and glasses. We decided in *Mad Max 2* that under these primitive rules there would be little time for sexuality and they wouldn't want kids, because a pregnant woman or a child is less likely to survive. A lot of people asked 'why did the warrior woman die, we thought there might be a love story?' – but she died because we didn't see her as a woman, she was just a character.

Max is not a macho character: he is tough, but without the sexually aggressive posturing of a lot of American movie heroes. Was that a conscious decision in creating an Australian version of that character?

I remember we made Max as young as possible in the first *Mad Max* – the actor, Mel Gibson was only twenty but I would have liked to have made him fifteen, it would have been even stronger – the whole point was that he should start out an uncorrupted normal sort of man in order to travel that distance to the other end. The hero who swaggers around and does everything good and rides a white horse and wears a mask is really a corrupted version – classic heroes are relatively normal people put into extraordinary circumstances. They often have one or two good attributes that stand them in good stead on the journey but they are not necessarily that swaggering macho do-good sort of person – they often don't even have a sense of doing good, they just know they are on some quest, but they always unconsciously serve the greater collective purpose, they bring something back to the community, they serve its rebirth.

In the movie tradition they are nearly always identified with sexual conquest – that is one of the ways we recognise the hero.

That tradition arose in the Westerns and so on but in our story we couldn't impose it. In wartime, in spite of war stories, there is not time for sexuality, though there might be rape and pillage. It comes down to much more primitive concerns: when soldiers come back from war there is a period of impotence, people don't come back with great sexual appetites. Then suddenly you get a baby boom, almost as a collective response to redress the wholesale death. *Mad Max 2* happens in a state of warfare and every time we tried to ask that question – we'd ask the actors, ask Mel, 'what do you think the guy would do for sexual fulfillment' – it almost became an irrelevant question. The marauders had a kind of recreational sex, they were crazy enough for that not to jeopardize their survival. I imagine that all those people who went away to start the new life would become very interested in sex once they felt safe, once they had established a place and saw that they could support children and a new lifestyle.

One reviewer remarked that in Mad Max 2 *you seemed to be much more interested in the bad guys than in the good guys who verged on being so wholesome and good as to be boring - how do you react to that?*

It is one of the weaknesses of the film. We believed more in the bad guys than in the good people - not that we didn't believe in the settlers' ideals, but the bad guys were just much more interesting. You can have so much more fun with the bad guys - one of my favourites is the Wez character, he is such a kamikaze type.

The presentation of the bad guys reminded me of the television World Championship Wrestling shows: you have the guy who comes out and introduces the gang leader, the Humungus, hyping things up ...

Pop pageantry - all good fun. It might have been a bit broad but it fitted into the logic of the characters - it is one of the techniques they have of surviving. But the wrestling - that was one of the guilty pleasures of childhood, sitting and watching all that stuff. It is a bit like Santa Claus - you pretend it is real but you know really, even as a little kid, that it is not.

Was the character of the gyro captain written with the actor Bruce Spence in mind?

No, it wasn't, though after Bruce was cast it evolved much more in terms of what he was doing because he brought so much to the performance. Collaboration with your actors is one of the greatest tools you have, and it is always so exciting to watch an actor who can take a part and make it their own and just fly with it - it is just the most wonderful thing to see. One of the worst mistakes I made with *Mad Max 1* was that it was such a tough and bleak story: it should have had more comedy. We did attempt more, but I found when we got to editing that I tended to cut the comic bits out because they were falsely imposed on the story. I learned that you can't force it, that it has to develop organically out of the story you're telling.

Were there many comic things in Mad Max 2 *that evolved on the set?*

One of my favourite bits is when the mechanics, Chris Graves and Steve Spears are talking – the Max character has just brought in the prime mover and they are diagnosing what is wrong with the engine and Chris repeats all Steve's lines. It was originally written for just Steve Spears to say those lines, but a relationship was developing between those two actors in their approach, and it seemed right that the Steve Spears character was so cool that he would have someone else do all his shouting for him, so that he works to maximum efficiency. So that thought 'why doesn't he repeat the lines?' came spontaneously, and they did it on the first take and it stayed that way. Then it so happened that there was an extra between the two of them and we said to him at the beginning of one of the takes 'why don't you watch the exchange like a ping pong match', and now when I see the film I watch the extra and find him hilarious. That's an example of something coming on the set that you can never conceive beforehand.

The dog provides some important comic elements too – there is a wonderful moment where the dog is holding the trigger of the gun that is pointed at Bruce Spence and a rabbit goes past.

That is partly casting too – he was a funny dog, very undisciplined. We wanted a blue heeler – actually we wanted a three-legged dog, but no one who has a three-legged dog and wants to preserve it would let us take their dog for three months. So we went with Dale Aspin, the animal trainer on the film, to the RSPCA's largest pound and went through the agonising process of picking a dog from death row. He was one of many that we saw – he came up and dropped a pebble at our feet and within seconds taught us a game where we'd kick the stone away and he would bring it back and put it at our feet. He coached us in his little game and we saw that he was obsessed with stones so Dale realised very astutely that we could get him to look in any direction we wanted just by holding up a pebble. After putting him through the basic training of 'sit here' and 'stay', it was a matter of putting him in position and letting him behave naturally. The only thing we couldn't get him to do was growl, until we realised that one of the crew members had a dog to which our star dog took an aversion. Every time he saw this dog he would start growling so we would hold the other dog up behind the camera in those scenes. It took us a while to learn that – most work with animals is observing their idiosyncracies and working that into what you are trying to do.

What happened to the dog afterwards – I hope he didn't go back to death row?
Yes he did. No, not really. The biggest problem was that everyone wanted to take him home. In the end Dale won him. The other funny thing that happened was that to get a dog out of the RSPCA you have to have them desexed, but with that kind of dog the testicles are very prominent and it would have looked awful – I mean, who would bother to desex a dog in that primitive world? So Terry Hayes prevailed on the RSPCA and they very kindly gave him a vasectomy. The dog, not Terry.

Did you try and time comic moments to occur at particular points in the film?
I think it is a real mistake to be that mechanical about it, the audience detects that contrivance. The thing I most want to do is comedy, true comedies. I can remember going to the movies as a kid and not being able to listen to the next line because the audience was laughing so hard and feeling sore because you are laughing so much – that is what I mean by comedy. Interestingly enough, films that give you that experience come very rarely – you can count on the fingers of one hand the number of films over the past 40 years that actually do that. If you watch a Buster Keaton film, even with a modern audience, or a Harold Lloyd you will get that response. The Marx Brothers do it, W. C. Fields, even though his rhythms were different, and Woody Allen does that to me in his earlier films. For me the test of a good film is one that on repeat viewing has the same effect that it had the first time, and films like Woody Allen's *Play It Again Sam* and Billy Wilder's *Some Like It Hot* give you that no matter how many times you watch them. It's such a fragile thing: I wouldn't dare do a comedy for a long time, but I certainly hope to do it eventually.

The Feral Kid in Mad Max 2 *is terrific – where did you find him?*
The little boy is Emil Minty. We worked with him for three months

during the shooting in cold, arduous conditions, and he was wonderful – normally precocious kids get to grate on you, but he didn't, we just fell more in love with him as time went on. He just walked in at a casting session and was a great little natural actor and very professional. The character came out of the Vietnamese street urchins – we used some documentary footage of Vietnam at the start because we begin in 1972. Those kids grow up with war being an absolutely natural state, as natural as the birds and the bees, yet they survive with the normal optimism and innocence of children. Like this character – he's tough, he kills people, he runs around with dogs, and yet still has that joy that kids have. We liked that character.

Were you aiming for a particular look with the lighting?
It was all exteriors, even the interiors were only inside a tent or a nissan hut. On a film like *Mad Max 2* you don't have a choice about things like shooting only at a special time of day. The horror for someone like Dean Semmler, our director of photography, is that you just don't have any choice: whatever light the great gaffer in the sky provides you have to go with and we even shot during rain. Joe Dante, one of the directors I worked with in America who had worked with Roger Corman, said you can always tell a low-budget film when you see a lot of scenes that are shot at sunset, which are not meant to be, because you are fighting time and shooting till the last minute. Several shots of *Mad Max 2* were filmed well after the sun had gone down, with just a last little glow in the sky: the high-speed lenses would come out and we would have lights put on – we were using every little bit of light we had, and being winter we had relatively limited light. If you look at the end chase you will notice how many sunset shots there are that bear no relation to the logic of the chase – I find it quite beautiful to see the golden glow through the dust on some of the shots, but it makes no sense.

The New Yorker *film critic, Pauline Kael, said in her review that she felt that you had thrown away the irony at the end of the film – Max has got the truck through that incredible chase only to find that he was in fact a decoy and the real prize is somewhere else altogether. The irony is acknowledged I suppose, in the smile that's exchanged between Max and the gyro captain.*

That is one of my favourite moments in the film. For me, that moment when Max watches the sand trickling from the truck is probably the pivotal point for him in the film, when he suddenly realises the irony that no man operates entirely by himself, that like it or not he is part of the collective. He thinks he is being entirely self-serving but there are greater purposes than an individual life, and that realisation is the first rekindling of his humanity. Without being too fancy about it, that is when Max begins to be, in the classic sense, heroic.

His reaction is very understated – there's something very Australian about that, which is something American viewers might not pick up on.

It is the first time in the whole film that Max even smiles. I love Mel Gibson's performance there – in spite of everything, he has no choice but to crack a tentative little smile, and it is definitely there. I would say that most people would pick that up fairly strongly – it is always a question of tone and balance and I don't think it should have been more underlined. There are other bits in the film that make me cringe but I love that bit. If he suddenly changed gear and started laughing like crazy it would not sit with that character. There is diminishing enjoyment of weaker shots in a film, where your mind goes into neutral, but there are some moments – and hopefully if I continue to make films there will be more and more of them – which even after watching them over and over again on the editing machines never fail to produce the same response, and for me that is one of those moments.

The music in Mad Max 2 *is a classic orchestral score – why did you decide to use lots of strings?*

A lot of people have said that it needs a rock score, that the *Mad Max* films are really visual rock and roll – we get that comment a lot in Europe and America. It sort of makes sense, except that rock and roll is not incidental music, it has its own structure and form and it has rarely been used well in films, other than films which are directly about rock and roll. Traditional scores of the kind that Brian May writes work synergistically with the film. *Mad Max* is clearly traditional filmmaking: it needs a score that works organically as part of the film and the best way you can do that is to use a classic symphonic score. There was never any doubt on either film about doing it that way.

Do you enjoy watching your films?
No, I don't. I enjoy some moments but as for the whole film, I'm getting to the stage where you couldn't even drag me in to see *Mad Max 2.* I think that happens to most filmmakers – you want to go on and think about new things. I have tried a couple of times to go back and see *Mad Max 1* but every time I have chickened out.

The   Dismissal

In 1982 you organised a collaboration between five directors on The Dismissal, *a television series about the sacking of the Australian Labor government in the constitutional crisis of 1975. Did you act as a producer in a day-to-day way?*
No, Terry Hayes, the writer, was the producer. Byron Kennedy and myself were executive producers, we financed it, and I worked basically as a director. The opportunity to collaborate with other directors was wonderful – there is so much to learn, film is such a new language and it's changing before our eyes – it will have changed and be gone before we know about it – so the more there is of this sort of thing, the more people try to understand the process on a basic craft level, the better. Every director has different ways of working – some work in similar ways to you, others don't, but you learn from everybody. On *The Dismissal* I don't think George Ogilvie had been anywhere near a camera, and yet we all learnt an enormous amount from him.

How closely did you work with the other directors?
We all worked together. There was a workshop for two weeks, which was very successful for directors, actors, everyone – because we were all intimidated by the subject matter, scared shitless of it. All five directors were there: at the beginning it was more group work and listening – many of the participants in the events of 1975 came and talked to us – then it differentiated out, and one director would take one of the actors and do individual work on the character. Make-up and wardrobe were involved at that stage too. The workshops weren't structured in the sense of normal rehearsal, it was more a question of

preparation. George Ogilvie, who oversaw the workshops, used this wonderful word 'seepage': it is all seeping into you, you attack it on many fronts, and come out with the group having, almost by osmosis, developed a collective focus towards the work. If there is no focus – no sense of everyone working towards the same result – the final product is diffuse and the audience is left stranded.

How had you felt about those events at the time?
I remembered it in the same way as when Kennedy was assassinated. I was stunned like everyone else, no matter where they stood politically. There was a great sense of outrage at the unfairness of it all: I was more politicized than I have ever been during that election and I was absolutely dismayed that Whitlam lost. In general I've been one of those people who like to think of themselves as staying outside the political process and observing it. We are amused by it or bemused by it and see ourselves as too dignified to get involved – and yet somehow of course we *are* all involved. I remember being very angry in 1975, yet when we did the series I felt more sad than angry. It seemed more a tragedy for everybody involved, and particularly for us, for Australia, than something to take sides on.

Did meeting the politicians during the workshop and studying the TV broadcasts change your views of the events or the people?
It demystified politicians for me – I saw them much more as people who are struggling with life the same as all of us. I had a sense that politicians are not as powerful as we sometimes think they are – they have pageantry that we might confuse with power but very few of them ever have the opportunity of being constructively powerful or creative. I came to see the Labor Prime Minister Gough Whitlam as a typical tragic figure, a classically Shakespearean flawed figure – he remained a little larger than life. And we were taken aback by the sincerity of Jim Cairns, who had been the Treasurer, and Junie Morosi, his secretary, though I had started out very suspicious of Morosi. Malcolm Fraser (who led the conservative Liberal Party) we saw as a much more subtle man than we had imagined, and far more astute than Whitlam as a politician. We think of Fraser as a haughty man who had had very little to do with the people, but he read not only the Australian public but those around him and his enemies with great skill. He had great insight

into Kerr, the Governor General, and his reading of Whitlam was superb, far better than Whitlam ever read Fraser or Kerr. Whitlam saw himself as a visionary and was great in that regard – however it blinkered his view of the close play.

Filming The Dismissal *must have been a real change of pace for you – the material and the treatment of it are so unlike the* Mad Max *films. Was it a very different experience?*
Yes, it was the first time I came in under schedule. The difference between the *Mad Max* films and *The Dismissal* was pyrotechnics versus performance. In the *Mad Max* films there is not much scope for performance. Mel Gibson is going to be one of the great actors as years mature him but with those films he doesn't have very much acting to do. *The Dismissal* was all performance oriented, and to work with those very senior actors in Australia was terrific. In the end what matters most is the performance, and how it serves the story – everything else should be subservient to that. The biggest problem I had on *The Dismissal* was in keeping the camera still: if you are insecure about a scene you tend to jazz it up with camera movements or doing something a little flashy – and I tend to be insecure about most scenes. But if you look at some of the master directors like John Ford, you see that after a while they become so confident they just keep the camera still and simply let the scenes play themselves.

You talk about the Mad Max *films being montage films where the emphasis is on editing, the juxtaposition of shots and so on, but* The Dismissal *is much less like that.*
Yes, it is more to do with the mise en scène, setting up behaviour and letting the camera observe. There were much longer takes – scenes would go on for minutes and minutes whereas in action-type films like *Mad Max* the shots are all short, and the pacing is pretty frenetic. That means you have to know exactly where you are to have any sense of performance – in a sense the action films are tougher films for an actor, because they can be so boring. They are even boring for a director: you spend three hours in a morning setting up a stunt and then you say 'action' and two seconds later 'cut' and it is all over. Then you have to go on and climb up to the next setup – they are very frustrating and arduous films to do.

REFLECTING   ON   DIRECTING

The   Role   of   the   Director:
Co-operation   or   Control

*People often comment on how egalitarian Australian film sets
are. But Uri Windt, who was secretary of Actors' Equity, has
commented that while that might be superficially true, it does
not interfere with the rigidly hierarchical command structure of a
movie. How do you feel about the role of director as the boss?*
If anyone runs the set it is the first assistant director. In terms of
management and people moving, he is really the boss and then there is
the production manager or the unit manager. That system exists to
carry out certain functions, and the director is the person who has
creative control of the film, who organises the creative elements. So
you are talking about three different jobs, each serving and interacting
with the other. It is not necessarily that the director is overall boss – it is
not a function of power, it is a function of organisation.

Don't bosses always say that?
There are moments as a director when you do feel ridiculously
powerful but they are the odd moments. For instance, we had
lightning as part of the special effects on *The Twilight Zone,* which I
worked on recently in Hollywood. I would snap my fingers and say
'lightning' and the lightning would flash. That was funny to do. One
of the great things about Australian crews is that they are very
democratic compared to, say, English crews – there was an English
director working in Australia who insisted that everyone call him 'sir'
and the crew rebelled by calling each other 'sir'.

But filmmaking is essentially an organic process in which all the
elements are interactive. It's like that question some people are still
grappling with – is film a business, a craft, or an art? The very
question indicates that people don't understand the process – it is
organic, to deny one of those at the expense of any other is to deny
what film is, and when one dominates, it fails. Then there is the
perennial question, a very forlorn question, I think: is it the writer
who is the creator, is it the director, or are films made in
post-production? It is all of them, each is just as important because

they are part of the same process. Whenever you bring a writer into contact with the director, or the director with the producer, or the producer with a studio, automatically people mark out their territory and adversary relationships result. It's tragic because everyone is right. We are all grappling with the same problems in making the drama work and if you don't face these problems in the writing then you have to face them on the set, if you don't solve the problems on the set then you are going to have to solve them in post-production, and if you don't face them in post-production then the audience is going to have to solve them for you and you are in real trouble. It is a problem if you are only writing, only directing, or only producing or cutting or distributing – you don't see the filmmaking process organically. That is why I think there will be a tendency towards what I call 'boutique filmmaking', where you must be a generalist to do coherent work.

I wondered if your medical training had an influence – doctors learn very early the habit of command, of dominance.
That's only because I was in the role of doctor. When someone goes to the doctor as a patient there is a definite ritual that automatically gives you authority. On Joe Dante's episode of *The Twilight Zone* I had to bring a prop over; I became the props man for ten minutes. So the role I had was completely different, and I found myself running to take the prop over because they were absolutely sweating on it. It depends on the role – certain roles give you authority.

There is a real leadership dimension to the director's position in a film crew which people handle more or less gracefully – how do you feel about taking that position?
It really rests in the work – if the crew can see that you genuinely love the work then they will respond and that is the best you can do to have people work in unison. If people perceive that you are cynical or that the apparent power you have is used cynically, then you can get into real trouble. But I'm amazed at how much people are prepared to help if they really think that you care. I don't mean all this bullshit 'let's all work together, let's be one happy family, I'll win your approval and you'll win mine'. It is a function of the work, of what is at hand. But if I

was with the same group of people and caught in the jungle and trying to survive then I don't think it would be me who would emerge as a leader.

Working with Actors

You've talked about the joys of the work a director does with actors, and you mentioned that you had done an acting course at UCLA – did that change your approach to performance?
It helped, but the best thing I ever did to learn about actors was to direct a short play, a little comedy with two actors. I worked with the actors through rehearsals then watched the performance each night, seeing how they dealt from moment to moment with the live audience, and how the performance varied. What I've learnt is that the actor and the writer suffer exactly the same problems and quite often it's the actor who can tell you the most about solving them. A writer who understands nothing about acting hasn't got a chance in hell of writing a good scene.

Can you give an example of what you mean?
On *The Twilight Zone* we were working with John Lithgow, who is a very fine technical actor. He amazed everyone with the way he could reproduce exactly the same performance moment to moment: we did ten takes on a one-minute scene involving an elaborate series of movements, and each take varied only in terms of my direction – he was able to reproduce everything exactly and make it seem real and spontaneous each time. I wondered how he could remember it all, but what I realised was that he didn't literally remember it. What he does is he plays it, he feels through the action to find how one moment leads organically to the next, so there is a continuity of performance. A leads naturally to B and to C, he doesn't jump to D. If it is not written for him in the script, it makes the actor's task much more difficult – if the writer suddenly jumps from A to D in the screenplay, then the actor has to devise something, and usually it is a false device, to get from A to D without going through B and C. That is the problem the actor has to face on behalf of the writer if the writer has not solved it himself.

You've talked about your love of chases, and the Mad Max *films have used chases, stunts and excitement very successfully. Do you feel your heart is with the action genre?*
No, it is in storytelling. Whatever the genre, the bottom line is storytelling. By that I mean the experience – the journey – an audience undergoes during the course of the film. That interaction between audience and screen is absolutely basic to all of it. And in all of that the storyteller's two greatest weapons are the screenplay and the actor's performance.

So you are interested in developing an emphasis on performance?
Absolutely. Because every special effect in the world is not going to make up for a bad performance, and a great performance will radiate through the worst technical jumble.

The   Director   as   Addict

You have used words like 'addiction' and 'obsession', words that suggest basically unhealthy states, to describe filmmaking – do you feel like that about it?
Yes, very often. Earlier on it was particularly bad – I could have been called a film recluse, in that I would want to spend more time in the movie theatre than anywhere else. For ten years, Byron Kennedy and I literally slept, ate, thought movies, to the exclusion of all else. We were obsessed with grasping the technical dimensions of it. We started with basically technical interests – but I think you break through that. From trying to examine film you begin to think much more broadly and I am very grateful for that. Through technology I got the Bucky Fuller view of life and through film I got the Joseph Campbell view of life. That is the healthy thing about film, that you have to have a divergent view of life, you have to look at every facet. When you walk onto the set you are dealing with what the sun is going to do today, what this lens is going to do, what this moment means to an actor, what the technology is doing, what the psychology is doing, what everything is doing. But I do think obsession or addiction is a prerequisite to doing good work, and that is often neurotically based.

Is it possible to be a balanced human being and a movie director?

Who can say? I am not sure I know what a balanced human being is. I'm not prepared to say that I am one, I think I do detect a more balanced life in other people. If you are really balanced you probably don't need to be a storyteller or a communicator – most of the things that drive you are healthy adaptations of a neurotic impulse. So I don't think you can excel as a movie director and not be neurotic. Ultimately, truly great work can only be done in great harmony, but until you get to that stage, it is probably the neurosis that drives you.

Can you maintain a reasonable personal life?

It is hard to examine these things – you might as well ask that of an accountant. Film is different in that you tend to be more peripatetic. That is the biggest problem, you don't have a sense of home. I only had one home until I got into film and now I have lived in so many different places it is not funny. That sort of thing can intrude on a relationship, but I guess they are not the main things, are they?

Well, they may not be the determining factors, but they can certainly be contributing ones.

Yes, that's true.

Going with the Flow

How do you feel about the question of preplanning and preparation? I recently read an interview with John Huston, a masterful and accomplished American director, where he advocates not having everything decided before you go on the set.

I think people often misunderstand this question. It really annoys me when people say that if you overprepare you risk getting locked in, because what preparation does is completely liberate you. If you are not prepared all your energies have to go into solving problems on the set. An example is Stephen Spielberg, who calls himself a 'born-again director' since *1941*. Before *1941* he would spend a whole day lighting and setting up, then shoot the next day, using very elaborate setups. It was the *Heaven's Gate* mentality. But *E.T.* was made in less time than *Mad Max 2*, it was done in 60 shooting days, its budget was only $9 million, which is the same as a high-budgeted Australian film, and he only rarely went to a third take. It's knowing you can use the tools, knowing what you can throw away and where you can jump, how you can modify things.

The attitude of 'oh, I'll be inspired on the set' is very lazy because it just doesn't happen that way. Sure, wonderful things happen on the set, but if you plan your film they are much more likely to happen. You can turn your film completely around if you want to – there is a terrific example in *Raiders of the Lost Ark:* there's a moment that always gets a big laugh when a warrior leaps out brandishing a big sword, preparing for a big set-piece battle, and the Harrison Ford character simply shoots him. What happened was that they were shooting on location in Tunisia, and everyone was sick with diarrhoea, they'd all caught some bug, and everybody just wanted to get out of the place. They had choreographed this elaborate sword fight and were about to start three days of shooting when Harrison Ford turned to Spielberg and said 'why don't I just pull out my gun and shoot him, then we can all go home', Spielberg said 'why don't you?' – and there is a great moment.

You've mentioned Spielberg several times, and you worked with him on The Twilight Zone. *What is it you admire about him?*
He understands intuitively how films function as public dreams, how they reproduce what we do in our dreams. You go to a movie theatre, you sit in a dark place with strangers and see things that can only exist in that theatre and at that time and they transport you. They are films more to do with the unconscious than with consciousness.

How do you feel about the tendency to make films like Twilight Zone *and* Raiders of the Lost Ark *that refer back to movies of a previous era rather than dealing with the world we live in now?*
Films are not real life, they are only the illusion of real life, just like any story – even a documentary film is not real life. If you want real life you experience real life – films are different, they are 'other than'. The great injustice done to the so-called 'film brats' is saying that they only live their lives through film. If you accept my view of films as

public dreams, to do with a collective unconscious and touching things deep down in us, you don't expect that they will echo the way we observe the world day to day: they have the illusion of being real, but they are not. You are dealing with things that existed not only in movies but preceded movies, forms that have been recycled many times –and we as audiences collectively need those stories and we somehow seek them out. So to say that the Spielbergs and the Lucases are failing because they are not doing something else is quite wrong – they are providing a kind of magic that is very important.

TV: The Medium is the Message

You used a narrator to frame the story in both Mad Max 2 *and* The Dismissal – *what appealed to you about that device?*
Terry and I had fallen in love with the notion of a narrator because it acknowledges in a very direct way that you are telling a story and we are basically storytellers. Secondly, a narrator is a bridge between the screen and the audience, between the characters and the audience. I think filmmakers are a bit embarrassed about using a narrator, because they think it's an excuse for not being able to do things cinematically. And if a narrator is used badly that is often the case –but one of my favourite films, *Rebecca,* begins with a narrator. When people started playing with narrative form it went out of vogue, but given that storytelling is a constant, one should not be afraid of using it. It worked particularly effectively in *The Dismissal* because the narrator there is very much a bridge between the events and the audience.

I could never work out what Marshall McLuhan meant by television being 'cold' and movies being 'hot' and I finally figured it out months after we finished *The Dismissal.* In movies, you are trying to enclose the audience in the experience of the film, to suck them up into the screen. But television, because of the physical constraints of the medium, tends to be something you observe, a little window into another world, while you remain very much in the world of your dining room or lounge room. A narrator bridges that, like a little person sitting on your shoulder helping you go through the story, and I think Terry worked this very effectively in *The Dismissal.*

Back to the McLuhan idea: two of the directors, Carl Shultz and John Power, who are very experienced in TV technique, tended to shoot in profile or long lenses with an observing static camera reinforcing the notion of the TV window. On the other hand, because I'm experienced only in theatrical movies I had a tendency to subjectify the camera as much as possible, using wide lenses, camera movement and tight eye lines. For example, if you are talking to me I would tend to shoot you face on, so your eye line is very close to the camera, giving the audience a sense that you are talking more directly to them. In other words the audience, my character, and the camera become one – not quite, but almost.

I found, too, that camera movement, which I do compulsively, is pretty well lost on television. In a theatre with a relatively large screen, you are moving the audience with the camera, they have a sense of moving from one spot to another, but when you are watching at home you have less of that experience, you are watching that little window moving, so camera movement is wasted. So broadly speaking cinema is a subjective experience, like being strapped into a flight simulator; television is objective, looking through a little window into somebody else's world.

Are you interested in working for television more generally?
To tell the truth I hate drama on television, *The Dismissal* notwithstanding. Television is a medium of lazy filmmaking – the production methodology has been corrupted by the medium. There's a sausage mentality. The filmmakers have to conform to that – there's a limited budget and a certain predetermined style. The only way television directors in America can get any individual flair into their films is to go out and get 'pirate footage' which is what Spielberg used to do. When he was doing *Marcus Welby* or whatever, instead of using a standard shot of a hospital, he'd sneak out on weekends with his cameraman and they'd shoot their own footage to give it a bit more flair. The television production machine standardises the product, because it assumes a standardised mass audience. That's changing now, with the increase in narrowcasting – developments in technology like the introduction of cable and video have allowed for much more differentiation. A program made for a narrow audience has to be much more sophisticated – if you're doing a specialist

program on chess, for example, it has to be much more sophisticated than if you include a chess scene in *Charlie's Angels*.

Serving the People

In what ways do you see yourself working for an audience – were you aware of working for a different audience in making The Dismissal *than in the* Mad Max *movies?*

One is always thinking of an audience. One little quirk I have when I look through the camera, is to imagine a little movie theatre, so in the bottom of the gate you see all the little heads of the people in front of you. You have to remember that whatever you see there is what people are going to experience in the cinema. The miniature audience I see in the view finder is always more than a hundred people, but there is no demographic profile – it is the kind of audience I become part of when I go to the cinema. But you don't try to second guess that audience: you don't say 'now this is *Mad Max*, so they want to see lots of car action because they are all kids,' and neither when you do *The Dismissal* do you think 'this is a bit up-market, let's put in some witty lines or imagine they are an audience going to an esoteric play'. You are always trying to be as lucid as you can and most times you fail at it, but you don't consciously try to play to an audience. The audience we were making *The Dismissal* for is exactly the same audience that we made *Mad Max 2* for except that the individuals who go and see them are different.

You mean you take the audiences equally seriously?

You must. A lot of people find it hard to believe, but I took the *Mad Max* films very seriously. The moment we start to get cynical, or start sending up the material we stop creating the illusion in the cinema, I don't mean the *Mad Max's* are without humour, but once you start saying 'it is just a car-action film, let's give the audience what they want' then you are in serious trouble. When we write a line for Mad Max we don't say 'let's make the line a little more straightforward or a bit more specific, because the audience that will see *Mad Max* is less literate than the one that will see *The Dismissal'* – you do what is appropriate to that story at that time, they just happen to be different genres.

There is a terrible cynical notion that many people have, that the audience only responds to trash in movies and TV. It is the single most destructive attitude there can be. And really you hear it most often from filmmakers, executives and critics – people who should know better. George Bernard Shaw answered them perfectly when he said, 'individually the audience may be comprised of idiots; collectively they are never wrong.'

Some people argue that trying to work out what the market wants through research is the best way of serving the audience.
I'm not saying that we don't do that, I'm saying that if that dominates your thinking you are in trouble. Certainly you ignore those questions at your peril – film is a business, an art and a craft, so that's part of the equation. You've got to know that in summer in most countries the core audience is between 14 and 24 years old, so that if you've got a film about Tibetan albino nuns and basket weaving, you'd be crazy to make a major blockbuster of it. However, if you're obsessed with Tibetan albino nuns and can infect others with your obsession – the financiers, the distributors, your collaborators and the audience – then go ahead. Likely as not you'll make a great film. If you were to ask me 'what is common to all successful movies?' I can only figure out two things: first, the obsession of the storytellers towards the story and second, their love of the audience. You must *love* your audience – want desperately to celebrate your story with them. No matter if it's the gentlest comedy or the darkest nightmare you're saying to them 'hang on to your seats folks – we're going on a ride!'

The Mad Max *films have a sort of Wham! Bang! Pow! comic book impact –were you pitching them at that youthful audience?*
I sort of knew my mother and her friends wouldn't like *Mad Max,* and we knew the audience for that genre is basically male, but we didn't say 'we must make it for young people'. It honestly doesn't happen that way – you don't start with 'how do we get as many people between 14 and 24 into the cinema?' You start with wanting to tell a certain story. With *Mad Max* we wanted to do a car action picture.

'Car-action picture' isn't a description of a story someone could be passionate about telling – what's the story?

I'm not talking about plot here – what I mean by story is the experience you invite your audience into. It's going to be different from the story you sit down and tell in words, or write in words. It's the experience the audience takes from the screen – the journey the audience undergoes in the theatre. It is experienced on a multiplicity of levels – mythologically, sociologically, psychologically, intellectually and physiologically. Truly great storytelling touches the soul, the heart, the mind and the body . . . .

But the phrase 'car-action picture' doesn't suggest any of those things.

Here's an example. Bear in mind I'm not suggesting *Mad Max* is great storytelling, but I'm just trying to tell you what I mean by 'story'. Part of the *plot* has a character, a road cop called the Goose, who is mortally burnt in a car wreck. Now the Goose is not only a workmate, but Max's dearest friend, so Max goes to see for himself that the Goose is dying – when he finally looks down at the charred mess on the life-support machines Max can't believe it's the Goose. So this is our plot for the moment – Max goes to the hospital to confront the sight of his dying friend. How do we turn that plot into *story?* How do we take the audience through the experience with Max using the language of film?

First a high-angle shot watching Max's police car as it screams into a courtyard below. In the extreme foreground we see an awning with the letters HOSPI-. We couldn't get the camera high enough to see the letters -TAL, but we figured the audience would fill them in and work out it was a hospital. There is not much emotional information here – just the intellect telling us we are at a HOSPITAL.

Next a tracked shot on Max as he hurries towards us along a long corridor. Now there is emotion here. Max is hurrying to something he just doesn't want to see. Approach/avoidance. So time is stretched out. His foot steps are extremely loud and the music is pounding like a rapid heart beat. The tracking shot is quite long. I wish it had been longer and if I had my wits about me I would have combined a 'zoom-in' with the 'track-back' to heighten the approach/avoidance thing. Now a reverse tracking shot quickening as Max pushes past three of his work mates to get to the Goose's room. His friends try to hold him back suggesting it's not a good idea to go inside.

Cut to inside the Goose's room as Max pushes through the door towards us. We hold his expectant face in close up for a long beat then we cut to Max's point of view and we see the Goose for the first time. He is just a shadowy form under a canopy in the only bed in the stark room. The respirator is making this terrible raspy noise. We hold a close up on Max's face as we track him slowly towards the Goose. The journey across the room seems very long. The leather in Max's boots is squeaking and with every step Max is getting closer to camera and the respirator is getting louder.

Now a reverse over Max's shoulder as we move towards the bed. Max's hand reaches out tentatively to touch the canopy. And bang! The Goose moves and something horrible seems to drop out of the bed. Max yelps and looks down. It's the Goose's hand – slid out from under the canopy. So here we attempted a shock moment. It worked OK but if it had been better the experience of the audience would have been acutely physiological.

Max can't stop now. He lifts the sheet to look down directly at the Goose. The moment is played entirely on Mel's face in extreme close-up. We don't see the Goose at all. We've seen his hand – that's enough. The audience's imagination will fill in the rest – better than the most brilliant special-effects make-up in the world.

So to some degree our plot becomes story. We go through the experience with Max. We know a little bit of what it feels like to go through that kind of ordeal. We are not just shown it. So back to our checklist – to some degree it works physiologically and psychologically, there's not much intellectual or sociological content in that scene, and as for mythology – well if Mad Max was a genuine hero of mythology the incident could qualify as one of the trials he would have had to undergo on his life journey.

I hope that all makes some sense. Storytelling is a much more complex and intuitive process than I've described. You can't really reduce it to mechanics. But it doesn't hurt to try.

With the phrase, car-action picture, we usually think of films that don't have those concerns, most of them have a primary interest in ...

In the pyrotechnics – and if that is all the *Mad Max* films do, well then they have failed absolutely. They have to do more than that, otherwise people will only go for the first week. They must do more than that, they must work on every level.

The First Feature:
Traps for the Unwary

Having gone into directing Mad Max *with very little experience, is there advice that with hindsight you would give someone in that situation that would make it less traumatic?*

There are so many things. It's a pity directors spend so little time on other directors' sets or working with other directors, because you face so many difficulties that you later realise are very common. You wonder why it rains when it hasn't rained for three months on the very day you absolutely have to shoot, or why what you thought was a great line when it was written just does not work when an actor says it, and why it is so slow and painful, and why when you see the final result it is so boring and you feel so embarrassed by it. But of course those things happen to everyone.

One of the most common mistakes of first-time directors – Peter Weir and Richard Franklin first alerted me to this – is to try and make every shot an A shot, to get perfection in every shot on a technical level, instead of seeing what the heart, the real importance of that particular moment is, and letting everything else become secondary. So if the lighting is not quite perfect, or the camera is a bit unsteady it mightn't matter, as long as the actors' performance is true or authentic. If you go out aiming to make every shot the perfect shot, you blow your time on the most mundane shots instead of using it to get that perfect pivotal moment.

But above all, I think the most common mistake made by a first-time director is slow staging; the rhythm of information within the shot is too lethargic. Richard Franklin was one of the first directors in Australia to use a director's chair and the crew he was working with pooh-poohed it a bit. But Hitchcock, for example, always sat slumped in a chair, usually in the same repose as someone in a movie theatre. What you have to realise is that the audience is concerned only with receiving stimuli from the screen, but on the set the adrenalin is flowing in a different rhythm and each moment is full of so much information. On the set you are watching an actor, you are also getting stimuli from the crew behind, hearing noise of a wind machine and so on – whereas in the theatre the audience watches that moment on the actor's face, unencumbered. So Franklin's theory, and I agree with him, is that the director's chair evolved less out of hierarchy than from the need to sit down and totally close out everything but what is happening there through that lens. In effect the director should simulate the repose of the audience. Then you may sense when the pacing is too slow. I've never heard anyone complain that a movie is too fast. The most often heard complaint is that they are too slow.

AN AUSTRALIAN OR MID-PACIFIC CINEMA?

An Australian Identity

Bob Ellis, the Australian screenwriter, has a good description of the differences between hero characters in Australian films and American films. He said that some of our actors, in common with some American actors (Humphrey Bogart being one), have a certain degree of self-distaste, a quality of being 'on to them-selves': he says that while Australians think of themselves as crims on parole, Americans think of themselves as Superman on furlough. Does that ring true for you?

Absolutely – you don't dare take on airs in Australia. Curiously, I think that is part of what Americans respond to in our films. Once you start putting on airs in Australia it is the beginning of your demise as an effective worker. It's connected to the 'tall poppy' syndrome, and I think it is more a healthy thing than a destructive one, particularly if it is applied to work. The moment work becomes static is the moment when a person feels they have got on top of the medium or achieved mastery. Film itself is just beginning and there are very few people you could truly call masters. And that certainly applies to the characters – 'crims on parole' is very apt.

How do you see the Mad Max films fitting into the recent wave of

Australian films?
They are certainly not typical. They belong less to Australian culture than they do to B-grade, movie-comicbook culture. But they are still essentially Australian – I was really struck when I went to France and Japan with *Mad Max 2*: people would say how peculiarly Australian it was. They'd ask 'what is it that looks so different about it?' and I'd say 'I don't know, we were just making a movie in Australia.' They said that if the film had been made in America it would have been very different. They couldn't articulate how and neither could I – but it's to do with language, with the culture, with the way the light is in the southern hemisphere, and so on. Even our cameramen come from a different tradition. An interesting thing happened to *Mad Max 2* in America (where it was called *The Road Warrior)*: it was basically treated as an art film, it could not break out of its Australianness in the eyes of the critics. It was not an art film but it did by far the best business in the art house cinemas and the big cities, and the kudos came to it as an Australian film. It got on the 'ten best' lists with all the more 'arty' films, and it won a prize from the Los Angeles critics – I've just brought back a plaque that says 'best foreign *language* film', which is pretty funny really. Its Australianness transcended its genre which nobody expected.

As an Australian have you ever had a sense of resenting the American influence on our culture?
I think anybody in any country tends to resent what appears to be outside influence. We tend to be very chauvinistic – look how people who follow football arbitrarily select one team and orient their whole lives around it. One of the good things about Australia is that we seem to be able to take the good things from Europe and America and Asia and often manage to avoid what is worst. If it is cynically imposed then you resent it, like when you drive down the road and see too many MacDonald hamburgers and Kentucky Fried Chicken. But that can be offensive to many Americans too, to see that sameness, that uniformity across their culture.

Your kind of filmmaking is strongly influenced by American popular culture – the comics and the B movies came from there, after all. There is a line in a movie by the German filmmaker Wim

Winders where one of the characters, finding himself humming a pop song, remarks that 'the Americans have colonised our subconscious'...

It's a great line. I think Hollywood *has* done that to the world, but I don't think there is a conscious malevolent motivation behind it. I think it has happened because they have been able to tell the kind of stories and provide the kind of experiences people wanted. The great Hollywood era of the thirties and forties resonated with people all over the world, and I think that happened because they touched what was common in all people – they understood then what Campbell is trying to tell us now.

Working in Hollywood – The Twilight Zone

In 1982 you spent some time in Hollywood directing a section of Steven Spielberg's four-part Twilight Zone movie. How did you get involved in that?

It happened almost by accident. Steven Spielberg had seen *Mad Max 2* and asked if I was available to do a film with him, because he wanted to do some work with other filmmakers. I was tied up with *The Dismissal* at the time but he said 'why don't we meet and say hello when you are in America next'. I got to America just as he was leaving to go to the Cannes Film Festival with *E.T.*, and the only night I could see him he had a meeting on. So I turned up to this meeting and there were the directors John Landis and Joe Dante and they were talking about *Twilight Zone,* a film based on episodes of the old television show, and not only that, they were filming this meeting for a television show, a profile on Spielberg.

Suddenly halfway through Spielberg said to me 'you ought to do one' – he is very impulsive apparently and I thought he was joking. He was, in fact, very generous. They had one extra story and it just occurred to him at that moment to do it. It was originally based on a terrific story by Richard Matheson, who is one of the three or four greats in science fiction – he wrote *The Incredible Shrinking Man, Duel,* and a lot of the original *Twilight Zones.*

I have always admired *The Twilight Zone:* the best thing I had ever seen on the Nazi atrocities was an episode of *The Twilight Zone,* and the best thing I've seen on bigotry, an incredible story about the trial of a black man in the Deep South called *I Am The Night.* In it, bitterness and hatred make the sky begin to go dark, and at the end there is a news announcement that the sky has gone dark over Berlin, over parts of Ireland, over Alabama. This was done in the late fifties, early sixties; it was just a torrent of rage against prejudice, and at the end Rod Serling comes on and says 'hatred is a disease but it is not a microbe; it is a disease in the hearts of men and you won't find it by looking in the Twilight Zone, you will find it by looking into the mirror' – very gutsy stuff. A lot of those things would certainly be softened and homogenized if you tried to do them for television today. And I've always had a great admiration for the way they did things in such minimalist style – they would have one set and yet the story never suffered, because they were so inventive.

Did you say 'yes' on the spot when they asked you?
I said 'absolutely'. It's not like doing a feature film, it's not that great a commitment, it's like going back and doing a student film – except it was on the studio lot – so for me it was very good fun.

Was the experience of directing in Hollywood very different from filmmaking in Australia?
The thing that I noticed in Hollywood is that everything is much more institutionalised. That's very much a double-edged sword, there are advantages and disadvantages. For example, I wrote a draft version of the screenplay, and when I finished I said 'print it up and anyone who wants to see it can have one.' But I was told 'oh no, you can't do that.' The producers have to get it first, they read it and approve it and then they show it to the studio – only very select people can get the screenplay and each copy has to be coded and numbered. It was the same with showing the rushes, or dailies as they're called in America – things happen in a much more ritualised fashion, and the conduct of the adversary relationships that emerge in the filmmaking process is much more institutionalised.

Francis O'Brien, the American executive producer of Gallipoli, *remarked on the different approach to screening the rushes – how in Australia everybody in the crew attends, and the director waits until everyone is there, where in America it is so much more restricted.*

It is generally much less hierarchical in Australia. My own Hollywood experience was not really typical: the crew I worked with was a young crew for Hollywood, and they were very impressive. I had heard terrible stories about union demarcation in Hollywood, and certainly there are old-school people who are really strict, with whom you can't even throw a styrofoam cup in the rubbish bin without infringing someone's authority. But I copped none of that on *The Twilight Zone* – they were the best of the *E.T.* and *Poltergeist* crew and it went absolutely like clockwork.

This is a very broad generalisation, but I think the camera crews, art departments, and so on in Australia are equal to the best in Hollywood. Where I found America much smoother was in the background organisation. Communications on the set for instance: everyone had a headphone with a little walkie-talkie system, so I had only to whisper into that and fifty people could hear what was being said – there wasn't any screaming or shouting even though we were working with six or seven wind machines and compressors. And I was working with what could only be called the best special-effects team in the world and they were just magnificent – never any down-time on the set.

Another difference is that the Americans are much more prepared to test things and get them right. Shooting time is very precious so they do a lot of camera and special-effects tests. And a lot more thinking is done for the director – for each unit of input from the director you get a lot more back. For instance, I would do my own story boards in Australia; on *Mad Max 2* they were such rough little drawings that the crew would look at them and throw them away because they could not decipher them, but I needed them. On *Twilight Zone* I worked with a marvellous young illustrator called Ed Verreaux who does all Spielberg's stuff; he literally shows you your film in three dimensions. I would go through the shots in the morning with my rough little drawings, and he would come back in the afternoon with them rendered into three dimensions, so I could see the film quite clearly and he became very much a collaborator.

So the biggest differences are firstly that the director gets a slightly cushier ride than in Australia, in that people do more thinking for him, and secondly that in Hollywood they are four or five degrees removed from error whereas we work one degree from error – on the edge. In the States they just can't afford to have things working by trial and error during shooting time. But those things are a function of a mature industry: there is fantastic experience in any given area, which can be used effectively. People like Spielberg are using it very well: he has turned the back lots at Warner Brothers and Universal into a little production house with a film school type of atmosphere. He has mostly young people working there, and like here in Australia it's a sort of cottage industry.

But the bottom line really is that there is no difference: there are good people and bad people, people who show great grace under pressure, and people who don't, whether you are in Australia or in Hollywood. The system is essentially the same at the technical level. Where it is very different is in the process of getting projects off the ground – in Hollywood it is much more difficult, and many more people are involved in the decision. Each actor of note has an agent, who has usually got the writer and director involved in the film, then the studio has liaison people because the budgets are so high ... There are many more people involved, so you need a very strong producer or director to have any vision or passion left in the film after all the politics.

You said your views of Hollywood had changed after working there – what sort of things were different from your expectations?
Initially I thought there was just one Hollywood, all the people in Gucci and gold chains and bright talk and dining in the Polo Lounge with agents and studio executives. But I realised there are about ten Hollywoods and you can pick the one you want to play in. I haven't met one serious filmmaker who comes on with hype and bullshit – I have been surprised each time and I feel rather embarrassed by my assumptions. You find what you need there – people think you must have an agent, but you don't; people think you have to go to all the parties and meet the right people and talk about 'development deals' – you don't. I haven't been to one Hollywood party: you don't have to do it, just like you don't have to in Australia. I think that whole game

is dying because it is not cost effective. There are many changes in the wind, because the technology of filmmaking and distribution are changing so quickly. At the moment there are only four effective major studios whereas five years ago there were seven and in general they are owned by much larger corporations – Colombia is owned by Coca Cola, for instance. And these days the studios function as distribution houses rather than as production houses.

How does Kennedy Miller plan to work with the American industry?
It is impossible to predict. For a time, as happens to every Australian filmmaker who has a film released in America, we were confronted with offers to work with major studios, but so far we've felt an enormous disinclination to change our style. Basically the way we have been working in Australia is completely different from what would happen if we worked in Hollywood. We would suddenly find ourselves working with entirely different methods because that small boutique cottage approach is very hard to get going over there except for the Lucas and Spielberg 'film brats', that group of film-school filmmakers, who have been successful enough to make their own terms within the Hollywood machine.

Will Success Spoil the Australian Film Industry?

Do you have any sense of why at the moment Americans are responding to Australian movies?
I think it's that they feel their own industry is a little jaded, rather than that we are doing anything that is particularly special. There is a newness to what we are doing and our films had, at least in the first batch, that quality of passion behind them. What is starting to happen in Australia, and what we have to be careful about, is that with the tax concessions, a lot of lawyers and accountants are getting involved and what they are passionate about is not the movie but the deal. The deal is important – an essential part of the organism – but not the nucleus.
Do you think those trends in the Australian film industry are an

inevitable result of the shift from public to private finance?
Not really. There are different problems with bureaucrats being the entrepreneurs of film because they are rarely by nature entrepreneurial kinds of people. The great thing about the first phase of Australian filmmaking was that the passion of the individual filmmaker had to go through the screen of the government funding bodies. Now it has to go through another screen and private investors must be convinced to put in their money – but paradoxically I think it is good that it is more difficult to get projects off the ground, because it really will test out the determination of the filmmaker.

But doesn't the shift of decision making into the profit-oriented sector increase the danger of those more cynical, commercially-minded approaches becoming dominant?
The essential thing is that if the individual filmmaker or organization is passionate enough about a particular film, it will be made by dint of that passion. It's not something you see by somebody talking loudly, it glows from the centre of them – and as crude as the money people's attitude is to financing or to business or to the technique of filmmaking, that passion somehow wins through because it is a greater force. I know this sounds almost religious but it is true. I'm not talking about a passion to be in movies, or have a particular career or lifestyle. It's not even the need to make a particular film, but to tell a story. If they are passionate enough about the story, about that communication, then they might say 'well, I can't do a film, it's too expensive – I'll write a book, or I'll stand on a street corner and tell the story to people'. So the bottom line is that it doesn't matter how films are funded. If funds were not available, people would start making cheaper films, or if suddenly there were massive funds and people started making bigger productions, it would only be those films that have that resonance that would work for audiences.

Your position seems almost fatalistic – but just now you were expressing some concern about the way things were going in the Australian industry. What do you think should be done about it?
There is an old saying from Hollywood that 'there is nothing wrong with the film industry that a good film won't fix' and it is true – all we

can do is make as many good films as we can. And I mean 'good films' not 'good commercial films' because a good film eventually becomes a good commercial film anyway – a good film can cut through all the talk and all the anguish and it energises everything in the industry. One positive step would be for budgets to drop – it is now cheaper to be involved in regional filmmaking in America than it is to be making films in Australia. It is cheaper to make a film in Texas than in Sydney provided you aren't paying those huge million-dollar fees to stars. I think there is something obscene about spending $20 million on celluloid: the result is so precarious – quite often the film might run indifferently for a few weeks and then be gone forever. All I could say, if I had to put out a little manifesto, is that it is a question of getting the priorities right: the priority resides in the intuition of the filmmaker and only then come the commercial needs of an investor or the ambitions of government to have a film industry.

How would you assess your experience in Hollywood overall?
My experience on *The Twilight Zone* was immensely interesting, in that I was able to see how the machine worked. But it is less interesting to me as a permanent way to work, because it is less organic – more specialised and compartmentalised – than our present approach to the work here. I am interested in examining the entire craft of filmmaking. The biggest surprise for me has been that the more you go on, the more you realise there is to learn. That's one of the reasons we've been organising a series of workshops for writers and actors and directors here in Sydney. It's amazing how really and truly little we know.

You have two choices: you can choose to keep it mysterious, and mystify it further – too often people who call themselves 'artists' play on that mystification, and that's one of the worst mindgames that goes on in Hollywood. Or else you can accept that there's so much mystery in the process that you have to apply an analytical approach to the craft to grasp any understanding of it at all. You can't stop and say 'OK, I've mastered the existing rules for telling a story in film' – because in six months time your rules are going to change. There is a wonderful axiom – 'the only thing permanent in the movie industry is change'. If you don't realise that the technology, the language, the audience and we ourselves are changing all the time, you have to rely on the mystery and never shine a light on it, never hone the craft.

We make a mistake in thinking that film is an art first before it is anything else. I prefer the Eastern tradition in which you first become a craftsman: a film director is basically an artisan working with a complexity of tools. The artisan hones his craft until he becomes such a virtuoso that he transcends the craft and becomes a master, and only when he is a master can he begin to produce that occasional thing we call art. If you look at it historically, the people we now call the great artists of film are those who were the first great craftsmen, and who during their time were only recognised as craftsmen – the Hitchcocks and the Fords and the Kurosawas. They were artisans first, journeymen directors. John Ford is the classic example – in 1939 he directed three superb films – churning out one film, leaving it to the post-production team and the producer and moving straight on to the next. In the occidental tradition people are designated artists first, whether by society or by themselves – and often that is to the detriment of the art.

AUSTRALIAN FILMOGRAPHIES

FRED SCHEPISI

Libido (1973) 'The Priest'

Production Company	PRODUCERS' AND DIRECTORS' GUILD OF AUSTRALIA
Director	FRED SCHEPISI
Executive Producers	JOHN B. MURRAY
	CHRISTOPHER MUIR
Screenplay	THOMAS KENEALLY
Photography	IAN BAKER

Cast

ARTHUR DIGNAM ROBYN NEVIN VIVEAN GRAY

The Devil's Playground (1976)

Production Company	THE FEATURE FILM HOUSE
Director	FRED SCHEPISI
Producer	FRED SCHEPISI
Production Manager	GREG TEPPER
Script	FRED SCHEPISI
Photography	IAN BAKER
Camera Assistant	PETER SYMES
Art Director	TREVOR LING
Music	BRUCE SMEATON
Editor	BRIAN KAVANAGH
Sound Recordist	DON CONNOLLY

Cast
ARTHUR DIGNAM NICK TATE SIMON BURKE
CHARLES McCULLUM JOHN FRAWLEY
JONATHAN HARDY GERRY DUGGAN PETER COX
JOHN DIEDRICH THOMAS KENEALLY

The Chant of Jimmie Blacksmith (1978)

Production Company	FILM HOUSE AUSTRALIA P/L
Director	FRED SCHEPISI
Producer	FRED SCHEPISI
Screenplay	FRED SCHEPISI
Based on the novel by	THOMAS KENEALLY
Music	BRUCE SMEATON
Photography	IAN BAKER
Editor	BRIAN KAVANAGH
Production Designer	WENDY DICKSON
Sound Recordist	BOB ALLEN
Casting Director	RHONDA SCHEPISI

Cast
TOMMY LEWIS FREDDY REYNOLDS
RAY BARRETT JACK THOMPSON
JULIE DAWSON PETER CARROLL ROBYN NEVIN
DON CROSBY RUTH CRACKNELL
ELIZABETH ALEXANDER PETER SUMNER
TIM ROBERTSON ANGELA PUNCH

PETER WEIR

Homesdale (1971)

Director	PETER WEIR
Producers	RICHARD BRENNAN
	GRAHAME BOND
Script	PETER WEIR
	PIERS DAVIES
Photography	ANTHONY WALLIS
Editor	WAYNE LE CLOS
Music	GRAHAME BOND
	RORY O'DONOHUE
Sound	KEN HAMMOND

Cast
GRAHAME BOND KATE FITZPATRICK
JAMES DELITT PETER WEIR
RICHARD BRENNAN

The Cars That Ate Paris (1974)

Production Company	SALTPAN FILMS
Director	PETER WEIR
Producers	HAL McELROY
	JIM McELROY
Script	PETER WEIR
Director of Photography	JOHN McLEAN
Camera Operators	PETER JAMES
	RICHARD WALLIS
Senior Editor	WAYNE LE CLOS
Sound Recordist	KEN HAMMOND
Production Designer	DAVID COPPING

Cast
TERRY CAMILLERI JOHN MEILLON
MELISSA JAFFA KEVIN MILES MAX GILLIES
PETER ARMSTRONG EDWARD HOWELL
BRUCE SPENCE

Picnic at Hanging Rock (1975)

Production Company	SUGARFOOT PRODUCTIONS
Director	PETER WEIR
Executive Producer	PAT LOVELL
Producers	HAL McELROY
	JIM McELROY
Script	CLIFF GREEN
Story	LADY JOAN LINDSAY
1st Assistant Director	MARK EGERTON
Director of Photography	RUSSELL BOYD
Camera Operator	JOHN SEALE
Art Director	DAVID COPPING
Consultant to the Director	MARTIN SHARP
Wardrobe Consultant	WENDY WEIR
Editor	MAX LEMON
Sound Recordist	DON CONNOLLY

Cast

RACHAEL ROBERTS DOMINIC GUARD
VIVEAN GRAY HELEN MORSE KIRSTY CHILD
ANNE LAMBERT KAREN ROBSON JANE VALLIS
JACKIE WEAVER A. LLEWELLYN JONES
FRANK GUNNELL MARTIN VAUGHAN
JACK FEGAN

The Last Wave (1977)

Production Company	AYER PRODUCTIONS
Director	PETER WEIR
Producers	HAL McELROY
	JIM McELROY
Screenplay/Scriptwriters	PETER WEIR
	TONY MORPHETT
	PETRU POPESCU
Director of Photography	RUSSELL BOYD
Editor	MAX LEMON
Art Director	NEIL ANGWIN
Production Designer	GORAN WARFF
Sound Recordist	DON CONNOLLY

First Assistant Director   JOHN ROBERTSON
Camera Operator   JOHN SEALE
Cast
RICHARD CHAMBERLAIN OLIVIA HAMNETT
DAVID GULPILIL NANDJIWARA AMAGULA MBE
FREDERICK PARSLOW MICHAEL DUFFIELD

The Plumber (1979)

Production Company	SOUTH AUSTRALIAN FILM CORPORATION FOR THE NINE NETWORK
Director	PETER WEIR
Producer	MATTHEW CARROLL
Screenplay	PETER WEIR
Photography	DAVID SANDERSON
Editor	G. TURNEY-SMITH
Music	RORY O'DONOHUE
Art Directors	WENDY WEIR HERBERT PINTER
Sound	KEN HAMMOND

Cast
JUDY MORRIS IVAR KANTS ROBERT COLEBY
HENRI SZEPS CANDY RAYMOND
YOMI ABIOUDUN BEVERLY ROBERTS
MEME THORNE DAVID BURCHELL
BRUCE ROSEN PAM SANDERS

Gallipoli (1981)

Production Company	ASSOCIATED R AND R FILMS
Director	PETER WEIR
Producer	PATRICIA LOVELL
Scriptwriter	DAVID WILLIAMSON
Photography	RUSSELL BOYD
Sound Recordist	DON CONNOLLY
Editor	BILL ANDERSON
Design Consultant	WENDY WEIR
First Assistant Director	MARK EGERTON

Lighting Cameraman	RUSSELL BOYD
Camera Operator	JOHN SEALE
Art Director	HERBERT PINTER

Cast

MEL GIBSON MARK LEE BILL HUNTER
ROBERT GRUBB DAVID ARGUE TIM McKENZIE
HAROLD HOPKINS BILL KERR RON GRAHAM
ROBIN GALWEY

The Year of Living Dangerously (1982)

Production Company	WAYANG PRODUCTIONS
Director	PETER WEIR
Producer	JIM McELROY
Scriptwriters	DAVID WILLIAMSON
	PETER WEIR
	CHRISTOPHER KOCH
	WITH ADDITIONAL MATERIAL
	BY ALAN SHARP
Based on the novel by	C. J. KOCH
Photography	RUSSELL BOYD
Sound Recordist	GARY WILKINS
Editor	BILL ANDERSON
Art Director	HERBERT PINTER
Production Supervisor	MARK EGERTON
First Assistant Directors	MARK EGERTON (SYDNEY)
	WAYNE BARRY (MANILA)
Camera Operator	NIXON BINNEY
Design Consultant	WENDY WEIR

Cast

MEL GIBSON SIGOURNEY WEAVER LINDA HUNT

GILLIAN ARMSTRONG

The Singer and the Dancer (1976)

Director	GILLIAN ARMSTRONG
Producer	GILLIAN ARMSTRONG
Production Manager	ERROL SULLIVAN
Production Designer	SUE ARMSTRONG
Screenplay	JOHN PLEFFER
	GILLIAN ARMSTRONG
Photography	RUSSELL BOYD
Camera Assistant	MALCOLM RICHARDS
Sound Recordist	LAURIE FITZGERALD
Editor	NICK BEAUMAN
Music	ROBERT MURPHY

Cast

RUTH CRACKNELL ELIZABETH CROSBY
RUSSELL KEITH GERRY DUGGAN JUDE KURING
JULIE DAWSON

My Brilliant Career (1979)

Production Company	MARGARET FINK FILMS PTY LTD
Director	GILLIAN ARMSTRONG
Producer	MARGARET FINK
Script	ELEANOR WITCOMBE
Based on the novel by	MILES FRANKLIN
Photography	DON McALPINE
Sound Recordist	DON CONNOLLY
Editor	NICK BEAUMAN
Production Designer	LUCIANA ARRIGHI
First Assistant Director	MARK EGERTON
Camera Operators	LOUIS IRVING
	PETER MOSS
Musical Director	NATHAN WAKS

Cast

JUDY DAVIS SAM NEILL PATRICIA KENNEDY
WENDY HUGHES ROBERT GRUBB MAX CULLEN
AILEEN BRITTON PETER WHITFORD

Starstruck (1982)

Production Company	PALM BEACH PICTURES
Director	GILLIAN ARMSTRONG
Producers	DAVID ELFICK
	RICHARD BRENNAN
Scriptwriter	STEPHEN MACLEAN
Photography	RUSSELL BOYD
Sound Recordist	PHIL JUDD
Editor	NICK BEAUMAN
Production Designer	BRIAN THOMSON
First Assistant Director	MARK TURNBULL
Camera Operator	NIXON BINNEY
Costume Designer	LUCIANA ARRIGHI
Choreography	DAVID ATKINS
Musical Director	MARK MOFFATT

Cast

JO KENNEDY ROSS O'DONOVAN PAT EVISON
MARGO LEE MAX CULLEN NED LANDER
MELISSA JAFFER JOHN O'MAY DENNIS MILLER
NORMAN ERSKINE
PHIL JUDD DWAYNE HILLMAN AND IAN GILROY
OF *"THE SWINGERS"* as *"THE SWINGERS"*

J O H N   D U I G A N

T h e   F i r m   M a n   (1 9 7 5)

Director	JOHN DUIGAN
Producer	JOHN DUIGAN
Writer	JOHN DUIGAN
Lighting Cameraman	SASHA TRIKOJUS
Camera Assistants	TERRY JACKLIN
	MARTIN BARTFIELD
Sound Recordist	LLOYD CARRICK
Costumes	ANNA FRENCH
Editor	TONY PATTERSON

Cast

PETER CUMMINS EILEEN CHAPMAN
PETER CARMODY CHRIS McQUADE
MAX GILLIES BRUCE SPENCE

T h e   T r e s p a s s e r s   (1 9 7 6)

Production Company	VEGA FILM PRODUCTIONS
	IN ASSOCIATION WITH
	AUSTRALIAN FILM
	COMMISSION
Director	JOHN DUIGAN
Executive Producer	RICHARD BRENNAN
Associate Producer	GRAHAM DUCKER
Screenplay	JOHN DUIGAN
Photography	VINCENT MONTON
Music	BRUCE SMEATON
Editor	TONY PATERSON
Art Director	GILLIAN ARMSTRONG
Production Manager	LYN GAILEY

Cast

JUDY MORRIS BRIONY BEHETS JOHN DERUM
CHRIS HAYWOOD PETER CARMODY
JOHN FRAWLEY

Mouth to Mouth (1978)

Production Company	VEGA FILM PRODUCTIONS
Director	JOHN DUIGAN
Producers	JOHN DUIGAN
	JON SAINKEN
Screenplay	JOHN DUIGAN
Music	ROY RITCHIE
Photography	TOM COWAN
Editor	TONY PATERSON
Production Manager	VICKI MOLLOY
Art Director	TRACY WATT
Sound Recordist	LLOYD CARRICK

Cast

KIM KREJUS SONIA PEAT IAN GILMOUR
SERGE FRAZZETTO WALTER PYM
MICHAEL CARMAN JANIS HAYES
ROZ DE WINTER

Dimboola (1979)

Production Company	PRAM FACTORY PICTURES
Director	JOHN DUIGAN
Producer	JOHN WEILEY
Script	JACK HIBBERD
	JOHN DUIGAN
(From the play by	JACK HIBBERD)
Photography	TOM COWAN
Sound Recordist	LLOYD CARRICK
Editor	TONY PATERSON
Art Director	LARRY EASTWOOD
Composer	GEORGE DREYFUS
Production Manager	VICKI MOLLOY
First Assistant Director	WALTER DOBROWOLSKI

Cast

BRUCE SPENCE NATALIE BATE MAX GILLIES
DICK MAY TIM ROBERTSON JACK PERRY
IRENE HEWITT ALAN ROWE ESME MELVILLE
TERRY McDERMOTT BILL GARNER
KERRY DWYER HELEN SKY PAUL HAMPTON

EVELYN KRAPE VAL JELLAY SUE INGLETON
LAUREL FRANK CLAIRE DOBBIN JOHN MURPHY
FAY MOKOTOW CLARE BINNEY MAX FAIRCHILD
PHIL MOTHERWELL BARRY BARKLA
MATT BURNS FRANKIE RAYMOND MAX CULLEN
CHAD MORGAN SANDRA EVANS
THE CAPTAIN MATCHBOX BAND

Winter of our Dreams (1981)

Production Company	VEGA FILM PRODUCTIONS
Director	JOHN DUIGAN
Producer	RICHARD MASON
Scriptwriter	JOHN DUIGAN
Photography	TOM COWAN
Sound Recordist	LLOYD CARRICK
Editor	HENRY DANGAR
Production Designer	LEE WHITMORE
First Assistant Director	ANDREW WILLIAMS
Lighting Cameraman	TOM COWAN
Camera Operator	NIXON BINNEY
Art Director	LEE WHITMORE
Music	SHARON CALCRAFT

Cast
JUDY DAVIS BRYAN BROWN CATHY DOWNES
MARK LUHRMAN PETER MOCHRIE
MERVYN DRAKE ZOE LAKE KIM DEACON
MERCIA DEANE-JOHNS MARION JOHNS

Far East (1982)

Production Company	ALFRED ROAD FILMS
Director	JOHN DUIGAN
Producer	RICHARD MASON
Scriptwriter	JOHN DUIGAN
Photography	BRIAN PROBYN
Sound Recordist	PETER BARKER
Editor	HENRY DANGAR
Production Designer	ROSS MAJOR

First Assistant Director   MICHAEL FALLOON
Camera Operator   PETER MOSS
Music   SHARON CALCRAFT
Cast
BRYAN BROWN HELEN MORSE JOHN BELL
SINAN LEONG RAINA McKEON HENRY FEIST
BILL HUNTER JOHN GADEN

G E O R G E   M I L L E R

M a d   M a x   (1 9 7 9)

Production Company	MAD MAX
Director	GEORGE MILLER
Producer	BYRON KENNEDY
Scriptwriters	JAMES McCAUSLAND
	GEORGE MILLER
Photography	DAVID EGGBY
Sound Recordist	GARY WILKENS
Editors	TONY PATERSON
	CLIFF HAYES
Art Director	JON DOWDING
Composer	BRIAN MAY
First Assistant Director	IAN GODDARD
Stunt Co-ordinator	GRANT PAGE

Cast

MEL GIBSON JOANNE SAMUEL
HUGH KEAYS-BYRNE STEVE BISLEY TIM BURNS
ROGER WARD VINCE GILL GEOFF PARRY
DAVID BRACKS

M a d   M a x   I I   (1 9 8 1)

Production Company	KENNEDY MILLER
	ENTERTAINMENT
Director	GEORGE MILLER
Producer	BYRON KENNEDY
Scriptwriters	TERRY HAYES
	GEORGE MILLER
	BRIAN HANNANT
Photography	DEAN SEMLER
Sound Recordist	LLOYD CARRICK
Editor	MICHAEL CHIRGWIN
First Assistant Director	BRIAN HANNANT
Camera Operator	DEAN SEMLER
Art Director	GRAHAM WALKER

Costume Designer	NORMA MORICEAU
Stunt Co-ordinator	MAX ASPIN
Composer	BRIAN MAY
Chief Car Mechanic	DAVE THOMAS

Cast

MEL GIBSON BRUCE SPENCE MIKE PRESTON
VERN WELLS KJELL NILSSON EMIL MINTY
MAX PHIPPS SYD HEYLEN VIRGINIA HEY
STEVE J. SPEARS

The Dismissal (1983)

Production Company	KENNEDY MILLER ENTERTAINMENT
Directors Episode 1	GEORGE MILLER
Episode 2	PHIL NOYCE
Episode 3	GEORGE OGILVIE
Episode 4	CARL SCHULTZ
Episode 5	JOHN POWER
Episode 6	CARL SCHULTZ
Executive Producers	BYRON KENNEDY GEORGE MILLER
Producer	TERRY HAYES
Scriptwriter	TERRY HAYES
Director of Photography	DEAN SEMLER
Production Designer	OWEN WILLIAMS
Art Director	STEVE AMEZDROZ
Editors	RICHARD FRANCIS-BRUCE SARA BENNETT JOHN HOLLANDS
First Assistant Directors	MARK TURNBULL STEVE ANDREWS COLIN FLETCHER
Sound Recordist	TIM LLOYD

Cast

PETER CARROLL MAX PHIPPS JOHN STANTON
JOHN MEILLON JOHN HARGREAVES
BILL HUNTER PETER SUMNER
STEWART FAICHNEY ROBYN NEVIN NEELA DEY
ED DEVEREAUX HARRY WEISS SEAN SCULLY

TOM OLIVER TONY BARRY NANCYE HAYES
TIM ELLIOT MALCOLM KEITH JOHN ALLEN
RUTH CRACKNELL CAROL BURNS
STUART LITTLEMORE FAYE ANDERSON
ARTHUR DIGNAM MARTIN VAUGHAN
MARTIN HARRIS VERONICA LANG
DAVID DOWNER LUCKY GRILLS TIM BURNS
GEORGE OGILVIE

PHOTOGRAPHIC CREDITS

Cover Carolyn Johns (*Mad Max 2/The Road Warrior*)

Page

(i) Kerry Conway (Sue Mathews)
22 Rennie Ellis (Fred Schepisi)
25 Film House Australia (*The Chant of Jimmie Blacksmith*)
26 Film House Australia (*The Chant of Jimmie Blacksmith*)
27 John Gollings (*The Devil's Playground*)
28 John Gollings (*The Devil's Playground*)
68 Courtesy of Peter Weir (Peter Weir)
72 Courtesy of Peter Weir (*The Last Wave*)
73 Courtesy of Peter Weir (*Gallipoli*)
74 Courtesy of Peter Weir (*Picnic at Hanging Rock*)
Courtesy of Peter Weir (*The Year of Living Dangerously*)
75 Courtesy of Peter Weir (*The Year of Living Dangerously*)
116 Stuart Campbell (Gillian Armstrong)
120 David Kynoch (*My Brilliant Career*)
121 Bliss Swift (*Starstruck*)
122 David Kynoch (*My Brilliant Career*)
123 David Kynoch (*My Brilliant Career*)
174 Carolyn Johns (John Duigan)
178 Carolyn Johns (*Far East*)
179 Robert McFarlane (*Winter of our Dreams*)
180 Robert McFarlane (*Winter of our Dreams*)
Carolyn Johns (*Far East*)
224 Carolyn Johns (George Miller)
228 Ian Whittaker (*The Dismissal*)
229 Carolyn Johns (*Mad Max 2/The Road Warrior*)
230 Carolyn Johns (*Mad Max 2/The Road Warrior*)
Carolyn Johns (Byron Kennedy)